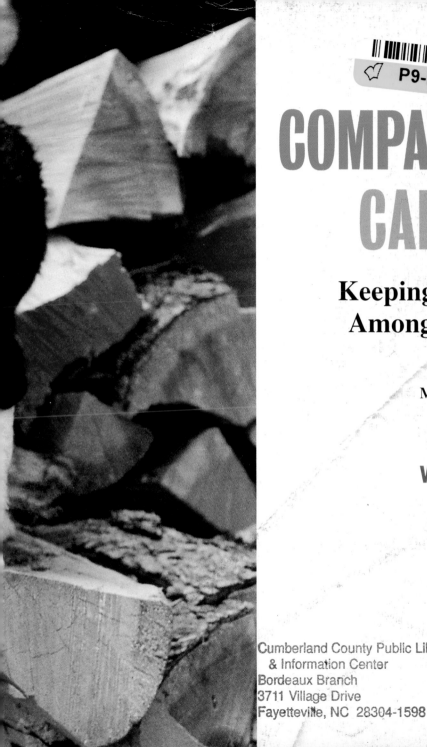

COMPATIBLE CANINES

Keeping the Peace Among Your Pets

M. L. Papurt, DVM

With full-color photos

BARRON'S

Photo Credits

Animals Animals: front cover; Joan Balzarini: pages 51, 109; Kent and Donna Dannen: inside front cover, pages 2, 3, 4, 7, 13, 14, 17, 18, 19, 21, 23, 25, 26, 27, 31, 32, 33, 37, 38, 41, 42, 44, 59, 62, 64, 66, 70, 79, 84, 85, 86, 87, 90, 91, 92, 98, 99, 117, 119, 123, 125, 130; Zig Leszczynski: pages 6, 29, 58, 67; Bonnie Nance: pages 9, 12, 47, 49, 52, 55, 69, 72, 73, 77, 78, 82, 88; Mella Panzella: page 128; Pets by Paulette: back cover; Marisha Riteco: page 57; Judith E. Strom: inside back cover.

About the Author

M. L. Papurt, DVM, is a graduate of The Ohio State University School of Veterinary Medicine and has specialized in dog care since 1962. She has more than 35 years of experience in dealing with problem dogs and their troubled owners. Dr. Papurt has counseled thousands of owners with problems relating to their dogs living in harmony with pets of several other species. She has written many newspaper and magazine articles concerning animal health issues. Her first book on dog care, *Saved: A Guide to Success With Your Shelter Dog,* was published by Barron's Educational Series, Inc. in 1997.

All inquiries should be addressed to:
Barron's Educational Series, Inc.
250 Wireless Boulevard
Hauppauge, New York 11788
http://www.barronseduc.com

Library of Congress Catalog Card No. 98-44323

International Standard Book No. 0-7641-0724-0

Library of Congress Cataloging-in-Publication Data
Papurt, M. L. (Myrna L.)
   Compatible canines : keeping the peace among your
pets / M. L. Papurt.
      p.   cm.
   Includes bibliographical references (p.) and index.
   ISBN 0-7641-0724-0 (pbk.)
   1. Dogs—Behavior. 2. Dogs—Training. 3. Pets—
Behavior. 4. Social behavior in animals. 5. Dogs—
Diseases. I. Title.
SF433.P36 1999
636.7'088'7—dc21   98-44323
                                                           CIP

Printed in Hong Kong

987654321

Important Note

This book tells the reader how to train his or her dog. The author and the publisher consider it important to point out that the advice given in this book is meant primarily for normally developed and socialized dogs of good health and temperament.

Anyone attempting to train an adult dog, especially one that the owner has adopted as an adult, should be aware that the animal has already formed its basic impressions of human beings. The new owner should watch the animal carefully, including its behavior toward humans, and should meet the previous owner, if possible. If the dog comes from a shelter, it may be possible to get some information on the dog's background and behavior there. There are dogs that, as a result of bad experiences with humans, behave in an unpredictable manner, or might even bite. Only experienced owners who have rehomed and trained such dogs should consider adopting them.

Caution is further advised in socializing dogs with other dogs or with children and in exercising the dog without a leash.

Even well-behaved and carefully supervised dogs sometimes damage someone else's property or cause accidents. It is therefore in the owner's interest to be adequately insured against such eventualities, and we strongly urge every dog owner to purchase a liability policy that covers the dog.

Finally, we advise all owners to be aware of local and state dog-related laws and regulations.

Contents

Preface

Pets enrich our lives. How much more lonesome is it for a child of working parents to come home to an empty house than to a house with a canine friend waiting at the door? How much more empty are sleepless nights without pets to talk to? How much less of an effort is it to improve cardiovascular fitness by jogging with a dog than by jogging alone?

Are two better than one? Most animal lovers believe so. There are several advantages to owning more than one dog and to owning animals of different species. Just think of the educational value, the amusement, the fun and companionship. When nobody is at home, the pets can keep each other company. Every member of the family can have his or her very own favorite animal.

Can you have too much of a good thing? Not if you exercise reasonable judgment. If you follow a few rules, each of your pets will add a special joy to your life.

Own pets that you really want, of species that you really admire. If you love both dogs and cats, there is no rule that you cannot own both, just because dogs and cats are assumed to be traditional enemies. If you like parakeets, you can own them even if you already own dogs and cats.

Keep only the number of animals for which you have time. Two cats do not require much more time to care for than one cat does. Twelve guppies can live in the same large tank as one pair of guppies. But five or six Old English Sheepdogs would seriously challenge anyone's spare time. Try to determine how much time you have to spend with a pet before you accept the responsibility for another life.

Resolve that you, not your animals, will determine how your pets act toward each other. Conflict is not a necessary nor an inevitable part of multiple pet ownership. If you allow each of your dogs to act as it pleases, you could find yourself living amid strife. You might be unable to leave your dogs together in the same room. Your cat could be spending all of its time under the bed. Your horse could be chased through a barbed-wire fence.

Pets are smart, but humans are smarter. With a little effort, you can manipulate your animals' behavior so that they will all be safe in the same household. This book is intended to help you accomplish that goal.

Chapter One
Dogs and Humans

"They're going to kill each other! I can't stand it any more—one of them will just have to go!" This harassed owner loves both her dogs and the dogs love her, but there is no love lost between the dogs themselves.

"Oh, I wish I could keep the poor little thing, but Taffy despises cats. The minute my back is turned, she'll eat it up." The kitten was euthanized at the city kennels because Taffy's owner allowed his dog to make the decision.

If the owners of these animals had understood the reason for their dogs' behavior, they could have resolved their problems easily and quickly. The owners could have taught their animals to exist together without conflict.

Dogs and Other Animals

All dog owners, raise your right hand and repeat after me: "I do solemnly promise to recognize that my dogs' actions are governed by their natural instincts. I will use these instincts to teach my dogs to live in harmony with humans, other dogs, and other species of animals.

"I realize there may be times when dogs' instinct will override their training. At these times, I will prevent my dogs from being harmed or doing harm to other creatures."

Instinct

Webster's Dictionary defines instinct as "an inborn tendency to behave in a way characteristic of the species."

Every animal is born with thousands of instincts of its own. Each instinct governs a basic behavior.

• The instinct to find and consume food. Unless they can obtain nourishment, all animals will die. *Eating is the strongest instinct in the*

Learning is most important in the behavior of a human; instinct is most important in the behavior of a dog.

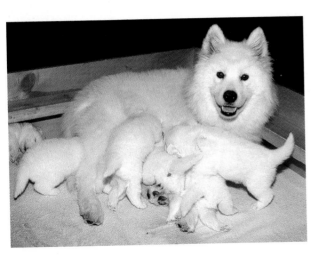

Samoyed puppies still depend on their mother for all their needs.

animal kingdom; since dogs are carnivores, their natural food consists of other animals. The instinct to capture and consume other animals is called *prey aggression.*

- The instinct to repel their enemies. Wild dogs must protect their hunting and denning areas from other wild canines if they are to compete successfully for food and nesting areas. The instinct to defend their territory is called *territorial aggression.*
- The instinct to reproduce their kind. All animals have a strong instinct to mate with others of their species. Unless they can mate and raise their young, every animal's species will become extinct. This instinct is *sexual aggression.*
- The instinct to live together in groups. Humans, canines, monkeys, and many other creatures are pack-dwellers. They choose to live among others of their own kind, both for protection and for cooperative hunting. This instinct is *pack behavior;* it leads to another

instinct, *dominance aggression.* The dominant animal in a pack can seize for itself the best food, the best territory, and the best mates. Dominant animals must constantly be ready to defend their positions from challengers in their pack.

Prey Aggression

Obtaining and consuming food is the dominant instinct of all animals. Prey species flee in order to escape being killed and eaten. The most prominent feature of dogs' instinct is the desire to chase, to grab, to kill, and to eat anything that moves. Prey aggression is vital to the survival of all carnivores.

Some breeds of dogs exhibit strong prey aggression; some do not. Humans have selected for the prey-aggressive behavior in the hunting breeds, but not in breeds developed for other purposes. Dogs without any interest in chasing even a tennis ball can live perfectly well when their owners supply their food.

Territorial Aggression

Wild canines (the progenitors of domestic dogs) establish a territory in which they hunt. The size of this territory depends upon the availability of prey animals that can be hunted. If game is plentiful, a pack of wild dogs can exist in a relatively small area; if game is scarce, the pack will require a large area in which to seek its food.

Pack members attempt to protect their food supply by driving other wild canines out of their hunting areas. This instinct, territorial aggres-

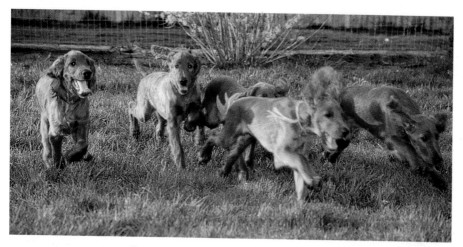

sion, is responsible for the guard-dog behavior exhibited by domestic dogs when they repel invaders from their property.

Sexual Aggression

Sexual aggression is an undesir-able, even embarrassing, trait in pet dogs. Sexual aggression leads to male dogs scent-marking objects and furniture in the house. Sexual aggres-sion does not create dominance aggression against other dogs and humans, but it often strengthens it. Owners of pet dogs are usually much more content with their pets' behavior if the pet is neutered or spayed.

Dominance Aggression

Each pack of animals has its lead-ers and its followers. Modern canine leadership is determined by the ancient method—the dog that can control the others by attack or by threat of attack becomes the leader. The behavior that establishes one dog as the leader is called domi-nance aggression.

When new dogs enter the pack, or when puppies reach maturity, they must compete for dominance. Even-tually, each dog establishes its own standing in pack society. If the dom-inant dog becomes weakened from age or disease, its position is taken over by a younger, stronger animal.

Leadership in packs of dogs is not absolute in every situation. The dog that is the fastest might lead the hunt, but the dog that is the biggest may seize the largest share of the prey. Canine leadership over other dogs may also be influenced by temperament. The dog that will risk snarling at the others may assume a more dominant position than is war-ranted by its size and strength.

Food aggression is one aspect of dominance aggression. Dogs' wild ancestors fought for a share of the prey. The strongest and most deter-mined wild dog took the largest share while the other canines in the pack had to fight over the leftovers. Modern dogs retain this instinctive

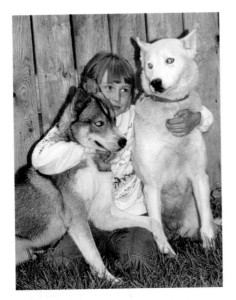

Kelly loves her huskies.

behavior. The domestic dog uses physical confrontation to take and keep possession of food and food-like items such as rawhides, bones, and toys.

Socialization with Humans

To a newborn puppy, its mother and its littermates are its entire pack. Almost from birth, puppies learn that Mother is the source of all good things—food, warmth, and attention. At about 14 days, puppies' eyes open and they begin to interact with

A well-socialized dog regards humans as members of its pack—either the dog or a human may be the leader.

their littermates as well as with their dam. By the time they are five weeks old, puppies have learned that they can dominate some of their siblings and that they must submit to others. They will have begun to establish their place in dog society. Before it is 21 days old, a puppy will recognize that humans are a presence in its environment. The puppy learns to regard this presence as benevolent or hostile, depending on the quality of the dog-human interaction. The puppy that is not familiar with humans by the time it is 8 to 12 weeks old will never be entirely comfortable in human society. The neglected puppy will be afraid of human contact; it may bite to defend itself from anticipated harm. Such a pup may learn to get along with its owner and even with its owner's family, but it will always be suspicious of strange humans and strange situations. It will shy away from people. The seriously neglected or ignored puppy will grow into a dog that will regard humans as aliens, not as fellow pack members.

- The young puppy that is handled roughly by *any* human will learn to fear *all* humans. Children who are allowed to treat puppies as toys rather than as living creatures may cause puppies to associate humans with fear and pain, not with love and trust.
- The puppy that is handled gently, stroked, talked to, held, and offered food will become the dog that regards the human race with unfailing love and trust.

Properly Socialized Dogs

Dogs respond to their owners and their owners' family members as if all are members of the same pack.

You can make the choice to be a follower. You can allow your dog to be the leader of your human-dog social group. If you make this choice, your dog will feel free to fight with any dog it regards a challenge, and it will attack any animal it considers to be a prey species.

Or you can make the other choice. You can assume leadership of your social group. Your dog will still have the exact same instinct to fight with other dogs and to chase prey species, but you will be able to control those instincts because *you are the leader.* You will be able to convince your dog that it is not permitted to attack another dog nor to kill your cat because you said, *"No!"*

Your Physical Presence

Most animals will learn to tolerate or accept each other without conflict, even when you are not present, but your physical presence may be required to deter conflict. A few dogs inherit such a strongly dominant disposition or such an intense instinct to chase that they may not be safe with other animals in your absence. You will be able to tell which dogs these are, and you will be in position to take appropriate action to prevent harm.

Abuse

You do not have to cause pain or fear to become the leader in your human-dog society. Whipping or beating a dog is *never* correct; it is not humane nor is it productive of your goals. You become the leader of your dogs when you train them correctly. *You should never resort to physical abuse.* When you have attained a position of leadership, your dogs and your other animals will live together in safety and tolerance, if not in affection.

Chapter Two
Breed Differences in Dog Behavior

The newborn puppy is not a blank slate. Every puppy is born with inherited instincts that will govern its behavior throughout its life. The vast majority of these instincts will become apparent only as the puppy matures into an adult dog.

At birth, the instincts that are manifested by all puppies are the ones that involve obtaining nourishment and maternal care. Newborn pups instinctively crawl toward their dam, their source of warmth and food.

The dam is the leader of her pups' society.

They instinctively grasp a nipple and suckle. They instinctively urinate and defecate when licked by their dam. Not until pups' eyes open at about 14 days of age do they begin to show other instinctive behaviors.

By the time a puppy is 21 to 28 days old, a few of its inherited behaviors become apparent. Four-week-old puppies will compete with their littermates for the opportunity to nurse and to eat from a dish. At four weeks, puppies demonstrate instinctive fear reactions to loud noises. Each puppy will develop species-specific behaviors and breed-specific behaviors over the next 12 to 18 months of its life.

Inherited Behavior

Some inherited behaviors are generalized; some are specialized. Even if a purebred Beagle puppy were to be reared from birth with a litter of pointer puppies and were to be trained by the same method used to train pointers, the Beagle would

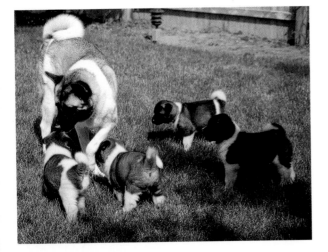

never learn to point. The Beagle could learn to chase game birds instead of rabbits; since its Beagle parents passed on the *prey aggression* behavior, the puppy will pursue any animal that moves. Prey-chasing behavior is *generalized* throughout all dog breeds.

If a purebred pointer puppy were to be raised from birth with a litter of Beagle hounds, the pointer could learn with its foster siblings to chase rabbits. All breeds of dogs inherit to some degree the generalized instinct of prey aggression; however, if the pointer were removed from the hound pack and given appropriate training, it could be taught to point birds. Pointer puppies have inherited the genes governing the *specialized* hunting behavior of prey-stalking (pointing) as well as the *generalized* hunting behavior of prey-chasing.

Experience and Instinctive Behavior

From the day of its birth, every puppy is influenced by its environment. Both its genetically determined behavior and its environment shape the actions of the puppy and of the adult dog it will become.

Example: Labrador Retriever puppies often have an obsessive desire to pick up and carry all objects, including game birds, but if a harsh trainer pinches the lips of a Lab puppy for biting down on birds, the pup will learn to associate birds with punishment. The pup may refuse to touch birds at all, even though its genetic heritage insists that it

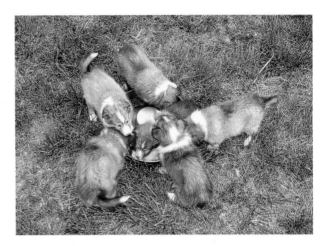

retrieve birds. In such a case, the pup's experience with harsh punishment has taught it to go against its instinctive behavior.

These pups are still too young to fight over food.

Development of Breeds of Dogs and Human Selection

The strongest animals of every species live and multiply; the weak become extinct. Animals do not survive long in nature if they are poorly equipped to find food, to avoid their enemies, and to rear their young. This is *natural selection.*

Humans select animals that have traits of direct benefit to humankind. Humans supply their animals with food, protect them from their enemies, and cause them to reproduce more animals like themselves. Even if these animals could not survive in nature, they survive with human assistance. This is *human selection.*

Dog breeders have an enormous number of genetic variants with which to work. In no other animal are there so many physical and mental differences between members of the same species as in the domestic dog. The five-pound Chihuahua and the 200-pound Saint Bernard, the racing Greyhound and the Pekingese, the Rottweiler and the Pomeranian—all are members of the genus *Canis*, species *familiaris*. Though the size and appearance of each are vastly different, each breed of dogs was developed from the same few ancestral types of wolflike or coyotelike animals.

Differences in Breed Behavior

These three factors determine the inherited behavior of every dog:

1. *The characteristics of its breed.* Each breed of dog has its own personality. Before you get a dog, consider how the physical and mental characteristics of the breed fit into your lifestyle.

2. *The characteristics of its parents.* Even though all members of a breed will be similar, variations of behavior exist within each breed. There are bold shepherds and shy shepherds. There are noisy terriers and quiet terriers. The most accurate method of determining the traits that a puppy will develop is to examine the parent dogs. It is from the parents that the puppies inherit both their appearance and behavior.

3. *The characteristics of the individual itself.* Every puppy will not

inherit the exact same genes as each of its littermates. After weaning, the environment of every puppy will not be identical. The owners of a puppy have the opportunity of shaping the behavior of the individual.

An Animal's Strongest Instinct—Self-preservation

Every animal must eat to live. The instinct of self-preservation insists that all animals' first priority is to obtain and consume food.

The wild ancestors of our dogs lived by hunting other animals. In order to eat, a wild dog had to perform a sequence of actions: It had to find its prey by sight or scent; it had to pursue its prey and capture it; it had to kill its prey; it had to defend its prey from other animals until it could eat it. Every task for which humans have used dogs is an adaptation of the dog's powerful instinctive behavior to get and consume food.

Performing Specific Tasks

Most of the more than 300 breeds of dogs were developed on the basis of the dogs' abilities, not on their appearance. Humans selected the boldest, most territorial dogs to be the parents of their next generation of guard dogs. The swiftest dogs or those with the best ability to find game were used to develop hunting breeds. The most active and aggressive small dogs produced the terriers.

Not until relatively modern times was the appearance of a breed of dog a consideration unless the physical traits directly affected the animal's performance of its designated tasks. Only after the advance of civilization made some of these functions obsolete did the purely ornamental breeds come into existence.

Even though the immediate ancestors of many purebred dogs never actually performed a task useful to humans, their more distant ancestors did. An individual dog or puppy may be generations away from the hunters or guards that were their ancestors; still, the behavior traits for which the breed was originally developed exist in the dogs' genetic makeup. It is vital to consider how the original purpose of the breed will affect the way in which the individual dog will relate to other animals.

Seven Groups of Dog Breeds

The American Kennel Club, the largest registry of purebred dogs in the United States, classifies breeds into seven groups according to their original purpose

Sporting Group

This group includes pointers, setters, retrievers, and spaniels.

Pointers and setters are stalkers of prey. They stalk birds, their instinctive prey species, until they get within pouncing distance. Pointer and setter puppies instinctively "flash" point for a second before they rush forward to grab the birds. Later they are trained to hold a point until the gunner approaches.

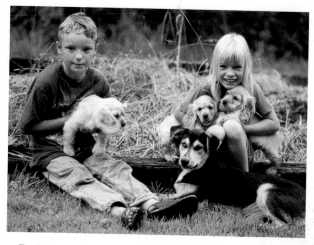

Retrievers and spaniels are chasers and grabbers. They find birds by scent, flush the birds into the air, and pursue them with vigor. Dog trainers teach retrievers and spaniels to sit when birds fly and to wait until commanded to retrieve.

Humans and dogs of all ages form social groups.

Retrievers are specialists. They are often required to stay near hunters until commanded to locate and bring back ducks that have been shot.

Dogs in the Sporting Group are very active and hardy. Their strong instinct to hunt can take precedence over obedience to an owner's commands. Many of these breeds require firm discipline to keep them under control.

Few dogs in the Sporting Group have truly aggressive temperaments toward humans or non-prey species. With appropriate precautions, most of these dogs can exist in harmony with other animals. Since sporting dogs were originally selected for their desire to hunt birds, extra caution should be taken when these breeds are around poultry and caged birds.

The genetic makeup of dogs is very complex; multiple genes are involved in the determination of behavior and appearance. Because of this, most of the breeds of bird dogs in the United States and Great Britain have actually evolved into two strains: the field dogs and the show dogs.

It is very difficult to develop a single specimen that can win both in the ring and the field. Many show sporting dogs have little actual interest in birds; many field dogs bear only slight resemblance to their show relatives. The disposition of the two types within a single breed may also vary greatly. The field individuals tend to be more active and less docile than the show dogs, a fact to consider when selecting a pet.

Hound Group

This group includes breeds that were developed to pursue furred animals.

Hounds are divided into two categories: *sight hounds,* such as the Greyhound, and *scenthounds*, such as the Beagle. Dogs of these breeds originally hunted in packs. Most dogs in the Hound Group readily live with other dogs, although many of them are relentless in pursuit of anything that runs away from them.

Sighthounds, such as the Irish Wolfhound, the Scottish Deerhound, and the Norwegian Elkhound, were developed to hunt specific mammalian prey. They were used in cooperation with hunters on horseback in pursuing and bringing down large animals.

Ancestors of scenthounds, which include the Basset, the foxhounds, the coonhounds, and the Beagle, were selected for their ability to find small animals by scent. Howling helped human hunters locate their packs of hounds, so these breeds were bred to howl when on a trail. Scenthounds probably will get along with other dogs, but usually will be noisy barkers.

Working Group

These breeds were developed to fill two functions: they were guard dogs used to protect people, property, and livestock, or sled dogs used for transportation of people and freight.

Wild animals establish their own territories in which they seek food. Wild dogs and many other animals protect their food supply by driving away other members of their species that invade their hunting areas. The basis of the guard-dog instinct is the protection of the food supply. Only incidentally does this instinct include the defense of property.

The ancestors of the guard dog breeds were selected for their fierce desire to drive competitors away from their source of food. Humans made use of this trait to use dogs to defend property, not only from other dogs, but from all invaders.

If a group of breeds must be singled out as difficult to maintain in a mixed society of animals, it would be the guard dogs. These breeds were intended to threaten or actually attack anyone or anything that invaded their territories. The guard dog breeds tend to have strong traits of territorial aggression and dominance aggression.

All these breeds are large, active animals with excellent biting equipment. Even though their behavior has been modified by selecting for more docility, guard dogs are the ones most likely to present problems to people who want many pets. Owners of guard dogs are well advised to consider the inherited dispositions of the dogs they own (and the dogs they want) before they buy.

The sled dog breeds, Alaskan Malamutes, Siberian Huskies, and Samoyeds, were developed for stamina in cold weather. These breeds can be a little wild and hardheaded, but only isolated individuals are truly aggressive toward humans or other animals.

Terriers

These can be scrappy creatures, and some may have aggressive tendencies toward other dogs. Their aggression is often a bluff—these dogs can be disciplined to accept other animals. Terriers were developed to hunt varmints such as rats, and are likely to try to grab small pets. Many of the terrier breeds are noisy yappers. Terriers bark more in company than alone, a fact to be considered before adding terrier breeds to a household containing other dogs.

Toy Group

These breeds are miniature dogs, designed to be pets and companions. They retain the instincts of their larger relations; many are active and alert watchdogs. Because of their size, toy breeds of dogs may need extra protection from other animals in a household.

Non-Sporting Group

This group is made up of all breeds that do not fall into any of the other AKC categories. The ancestors of these breeds performed many functions: The Standard Poodle was originally a water retriever, the Bulldog was used in the "sport" of bullbaiting. Most of the non-sporting dogs are relatively willing to exist with other animals, although a few may demonstrate excessive dominance-aggression.

Herding Group

These dogs include the collie- and shepherd-type breeds. Some of these breeds, such as the German Shepherd Dog, more closely resemble a guard dog in temperament than an actual herder of flocks.

The prey aggressive behavior of herding dogs is arrested at the chasing stage. Humans selected those individuals that chased other animals but that had a reduced desire to grab and kill. Humans then selected individual dogs that could be trained to chase livestock only under human direction.

Herding dogs are among the most responsive of all breeds to training. A larger proportion of obedience and

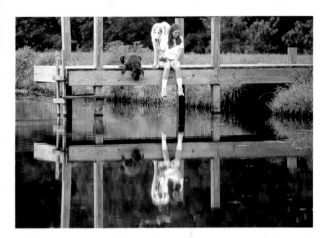

Dogs and humans share beautiful moments.

agility degrees are held by dogs of this group than of any other. Except for the individuals in this group that possess the aggressive territorial behavior of guard dogs, herding dogs usually are readily adaptable to a multiple-animal society.

A word about Pit Bulldogs. The United Kennel Club recognizes the American Pit Bull Terrier and the American Kennel Club recognizes the Staffordshire Bull Terrier and the white or colored varieties of the Bull Terrier. Neither kennel club tolerates any breed of dog bred for fighting. The dispositions of the Staffordshires, the Bull Terriers, and the American Pit Bull Terriers are similar to that of any other large terrier. Even if their ancestors were fighting dogs, this trait has been eliminated from purebred modern bull terriers by selective breeding.

Dog fighting as a sport is illegal everywhere in the United States; however, there does exist the fighting Pit Bulldog, bred and fought outside the law. These are not pure-breds in the usual sense. Their ancestry is composed of whatever dogs their owners considered to be fierce fighters. The true Pit Bulldog is intended to be aggressive toward other dogs, not toward people. Some of these animals are kept as guard dogs and encouraged to threaten or actually attack humans by persons who regard a dangerous animal as a status symbol. Unfortunately, it is not possible to tell by physical appearance alone which of these dogs are fighters. Prospective owners are well advised to avoid Pit Bull-type dogs of unknown origin.

Breeding for Appearance vs. Behavior

The prize winners in the earliest dog shows were those animals that the judges *knew* could do their jobs. Eventually, the more exaggerated physical characteristics became the standard for the breed: In a breed that was aided by a heavy coat, the individuals with the greatest coat would get the ribbons; prizes in a small breed would go to the smallest dogs; the long-eared hound classes would be won by those whose ears dragged on the ground. Modern breed standards of appearance—which often change—describe mainly a dog's physical characteristics and disregard its behavior so long as the dog's show-ring deportment is acceptable.

Chapter Three
Learned Behavior

Do you want to be a one-dog owner, or would you like to have the pleasure and companionship of more than one pet? If you settle for having only a single animal in your household because you fear your resident dog's attitude toward another dog, you allow your dog to make the choice.

If you permit your resident dog to act as it pleases, you will find it extremely difficult to add another pet to your household. If you do acquire another dog, you are likely to find yourself in one of the following situations:

1. *Your resident dog will be actively hostile toward a new dog.* It will exhibit *territorial aggression* and try to expel the newcomer. The dogs will fight whenever they are together.

2. *Your present dog will consider the new dog to be an addition to the pack.* Confrontation between the two will be caused by *dominance aggression;* the dogs will fight until or unless one dog is willing to allow the other to be the pack leader.

3. *Your resident dog will not be hostile toward the new dog, but will be unruly and overexcited by the presence of the other animal.* It will try to initiate rough, vigorous play with the new dog. If your new dog is a puppy, this might result in your resident dog harming it, intentionally or accidentally. If your new dog is an adult, the rough play might escalate into hostility and aggression on the part of either of the dogs. Even if they do not fight, your household will be disrupted by the dogs' vigorous activity and you may decide

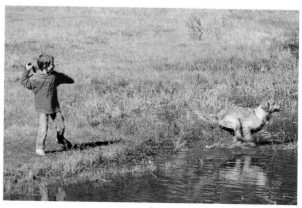

Retrievers are born to chase.

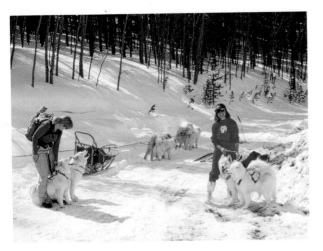

Arctic breeds inherently love to work in the snow.

that having another pet is not worth the trouble.

If you teach your dog that you are in control of its behavior, you can add as many pets as you wish to your "pack." The dogs will soon learn that they have no choice but to accept each other. They will learn to live together without overt hostility, without fighting, and without tearing your house apart.

Establishing Your Position as Pack Leader

When you are the pack leader, you can control your dogs' actions even in the presence of other animals. You can control your dogs' actions even when their instincts act to promote aggression against new animals in your society.

What does it mean to be a pack leader? Leaders can handle their dogs in any non-painful way they wish:

- They can comb and brush their dogs. They can comb the long hair on the dogs' hind legs; they can roll the dogs over and comb their stomachs.
- They can cut their dogs' nails and clean their ears.
- They can pick up their dogs' food dishes and bones, even when the dogs are eating or chewing. Leaders' dogs will never bite them nor threaten to bite them.

Leaders can prevent their dogs from engaging in unacceptable behavior such as attacking other animals *when the leader is present.* Not all dogs can be trusted to tolerate other animals when their leaders are not there to control them.

Use Gentle, Firm Restraint

Dogs do not understand the concept of gratitude. Even though you are the source of all good things— food, praise, exercise—your dog will not relinquish its social status to you simply because it is grateful for your care. A dog cannot understand that your continued kindness toward it is dependent upon its behavior. You must use another method of establishing yourself as the leader.

Dogs understand the concept of superior strength and determination. A dog's social position is determined by the willingness of the other members of its society to defer to its wishes.

Determination is a more important factor than is mere strength. A feisty

Pekingese can bluff a submissive Doberman away from its own food, even though the Doberman could destroy the Pekingese with one snap. If the dominant pack member appears willing to bite, the submissive member will back down. If the Doberman were not submissive, the Pekingese would not stand a chance. If the dominant pack member is the human, the dog will not offer a challenge. If the dominant member is the dog, the human might be bitten.

You can become the leader in your dog-human society only by showing your dogs that they must submit because you are *physically capable* of dominating them. There is absolutely no cruelty, no beating, and no pain involved in this lesson. Most puppies and dogs will not consider this lesson anything other than routine handling. Those dogs that resist the lesson will soon learn that their resistance is futile, that you are the leader. The few dogs that struggle against your handling are the ones that need the lesson the most. These are the dogs that will disregard your commands, and will bite you if they cannot have their own way.

Gentle, firm restraint is the key to the dominance of every dog. The dog that discovers that it is unable to resist your physical control is the dog that will be willing to defer to your wishes. The dog that realizes that your control causes it no pain is the dog that will be submissive but not afraid of you. This training is easy, quick, and long-lasting—in

only a few lessons, dogs learn to be submissive to their owners for life.

Teach the Dog the Submissive Position

When establishing dominance over a puppy, the mother dog growls and pins the puppy to the ground with her jaws. Soon the puppy learns to crouch down or roll over whenever its mother growls, without even waiting for the physical restraint. The puppy becomes submissive toward its mother.

A pack leader demonstrates its dominance over another dog in the same way—it growls. If the other dog fails to demonstrate submission, the leader grabs the other dog by the throat and holds it down. If the other dog submits to the restraint by not struggling, the leader releases its hold. If the other dog struggles, the leader may intensify its attack. If the other dog is strong enough or determined enough not to be held down, a fight may ensue. Leadership may pass to the other dog.

You can establish dominance over your dog by causing it to assume the submissive position, just as its mother did. Place the dog on its side. Hold it there until it no longer struggles to rise. When the dog stops struggling and accepts your control, allow it to get up and give it praise. Repeat this lesson until the dog does not resist being placed on its side and no longer struggles until you release your hold. When your dog does not resist the position, it has learned to be submissive to your handling. It will also be submissive toward its owner's wishes and obedient to its owner's commands because it accepts the owner as its leader.

The easiest method of placing a dog on its side is to push it into a sitting position, pull its front legs forward until it is lying down, then roll it over. Never grab a dog by its legs and slam it to the ground.

Offer no praise or soothing words if your dog resists being placed or held in the submissive position. Praise is for good behavior; resistance is bad behavior. Praise only when the dog offers no resistance at all. Say, "No! No!" if the dog resists.

Most puppies will learn the submissive position in two or three lessons. The average adult dog will offer mild resistance to being placed in the submissive position, but little resistance to being held there. Puppies and dogs should have one or two lessons a day only for as long as they demonstrate any resistance. When your dog recognizes you as the dominant member of its society, forget the submissive position and go on to other training. You can always repeat the lesson a few more times if you have a reason to question your dog's willingness to submit to you.

A few dogs will struggle violently and even try to bite when placed in the submissive position. These are the dogs that insist on dominating their owners. If you are to control these dogs' behavior, you have to change their minds without being bitten. Dogs that succeed in intimidating you into giving up have their dominant behavior reinforced. If you fear that your dog may bite if placed in the position, muzzle it until it learns to accept your handling.

Pay no attention to the dog that seemingly screams in fear when placed in the submissive position. If you give up because you think you are terrifying your dog, it will learn that all it has to do is to struggle and cry to resist your control. If you do not give up, the dog will learn that the handling causes it no harm. It will learn not to fear you in any situation.

Be careful: A frightened dog will bite just as hard as a resistant one. Muzzle any dog that you feel is not safe to handle. You can remove the muzzle when the dog learns that you will not hurt it.

Controlling Your Dog's Aggression

When you have established yourself as the leader of your "pack," you can control your dog's behavior toward other dogs and all other animals.

You can interrupt or inhibit your dog's aggressive behavior because the dog obeys the command: *"Down."* A dog that obeys *"Down"* cannot attack at the same time.

You can remove your dog from aggressive situations because it obeys the command: *"Come."* A dog that comes to you cannot chase another animal. When you have your dog immobilized in the *down* position or within your reach in the *come* position, you can snap a leash onto its collar and lead it away from the source of conflict and danger.

How can you establish this much control over an animal? It is time-consuming, but it is not difficult. Anyone with determination and patience can do it.

- Teach your dog that you are the leader with the use of the submissive position. You can convince your dog that you are a benevolent boss, but a boss who must be obeyed.
- Teach your dog the meaning of a few simple words such as *down* and *come*. Chapter Six will help you to accomplish this.
- Remove restraint equipment such as the headcollar *only* when you are sure that your dog is dependably under the control of your voice.
- Be patient and never take chances. It is worth a few more days or weeks of training to avoid aggressive episodes among your dogs.

Chapter Four
Will They Fight?

More than 80 percent of the time, your resident dog will readily accept a new canine addition to its household. After a minimum of sniffing and circling, most dogs are willing to coexist with other dogs without animosity. Approximately one dog in five will be actively aggressive toward any strange dog that enters its environment. A few dogs will fight to the death to defend their home territories from all invaders.

How can you tell in advance what will happen when you bring a new dog home? If you have taken your dog to obedience school, you will have observed its behavior toward its classmates, but not toward strange dogs on its home territory. If you own more than one dog, you know how each of them gets along with the others, but not if they all will accept a stranger or if they will gang up against one. The factors that influence dog interrelationships are controlled by the normal structure of canine society.

Age

A dog's puppyhood is over at approximately 14 months. From then until the dog is about two years old, it can be considered a juvenile. An adult dog is about two years old but less than 10 or 12 years, the time at which most breeds begin to look and act old. A truly old dog is one that shows signs of senility. This occurs at about 15 years old for small breeds, 12 years for large breeds.

Puppies are not often aggressive toward adult dogs. When you introduce a puppy into your household

The Mastiff pup wants to be friends; the Border Collie would rather hide.

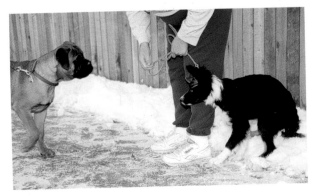

containing one or more adult dogs, you must guard against the resident dogs harming the pup, but very seldom against the puppy challenging the others. If you acquire an adult dog and your resident dogs are all puppies, the pups probably will accept the newcomer as a dog of higher social standing as befits its age.

Problems in persuading resident dogs to accept newcomers are most common when all are adults. The resident dogs may challenge all other adult dogs that invade their territory, so you must be ready to introduce your new dog in such a way as to minimize turmoil.

Sex

Adult male dogs are more likely to show aggression toward other dogs than are females. Male dogs are more likely to act aggressive toward other males, females toward other females. This is a rule, not an absolute fact. Do not assume that your resident females will not fight, or that your resident males will not fight with strange females.

Neutering/Spaying

Neutering a dog will not prevent it from fighting with other dogs, male or female. Spaying and neutering dogs remove only their reproductive urges, not their instinct to guard their property. Spayed and neutered dogs *may* be less likely to fight with other dogs; it is estimated that neutering

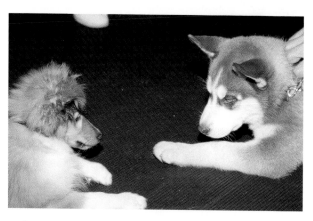

Cautious strangers.

reduces aggression in 50 to 60 percent of dogs. Use caution when you introduce a new dog, even if all of them are altered.

There is one huge advantage to neutering all male house dogs before they reach puberty. Dogs neutered before puberty (five to ten months of age) seldom develop the habit of scent-marking—squirting small amounts of their urine in many places to leave their own personal smell everywhere in their territory. *Every* adult male dog that is not neutered will scent-mark when a strange canine enters its home. Unless you do not object to smelly yellow drapes and sofas, have your dog neutered.

Breed and Size

Chapter Two detailed the influence of genetics on dogs' acceptance of other dogs. Breeds such as Beagles that were developed to hunt in packs are more likely to exist peacefully with other dogs than are breeds such as Akitas that were meant to be solitary guard dogs. Consider the purpose for which your breed was developed when you decide to acquire another dog. Be prepared to use stern measures when introducing two adults of the working or guarding breeds.

Size has little bearing on the inherited instincts of dogs; small dogs may be just as aggressive as larger ones. Size may influence a dog's behavior toward humans if the small dog has learned that its owner can easily physically control it; however, small dogs seem to have little fear of challenging a larger dog that invades their territory. Be careful that your resident Pekingese does not try to attack your new German Shepherd.

Six Behavior Groups

Group 1

These dogs instantly accept all other dogs, both at their homes and in unfamiliar settings. They rush toward other dogs, head high and tail wagging. They lick and sniff other dogs. They may institute play, but they do not jump up on other dogs.

Group 1 dogs may lower their heads, crouch, or roll over in submission to new canine acquaintances. Group 1 dogs never growl, although they might bark in excitement.

Almost all puppies are members of Group 1, as are about a quarter of all adult dogs, even though they may have had no previous canine contacts. If your resident dog is in this group, it will be easy to introduce any nonaggressive dog into your home.

Group 2

Group 2 dogs include those dogs that act friendly toward other dogs away from home, but are suspicious of other dogs in their own personal territories. In their homes, Group 2 dogs might approach a newcomer stiff-legged and with raised hair on their shoulders, but will be willing to sniff, be sniffed, and engage in play behavior within a few minutes. Group 2 dogs of both sexes may exhibit dominant mounting behavior and may growl at each other, but are unlikely to actually attack one another.

Group 3

Dogs in this group act much as do dogs in Group 2, except that they do not engage in play activity with strange dogs. Group 3 dogs choose to ignore or avoid newcomers. They may stalk away or slink into a corner and lie down; they may growl or snap if a new dog insists on bothering them. Never let your new puppy pester your Group 3 resident, or your puppy may receive a serious bite.

Group 4

These dogs actually challenge strange dogs at home, although they will usually ignore them on the street or in obedience classes. Group 4 dogs will approach other dogs in their homes with raised hackles and bared teeth, and may attack unless

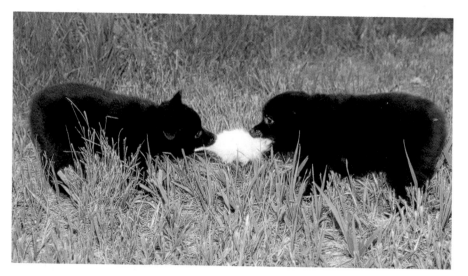

These Schipperke pups each want the same "prey object."

the newcomers act submissive. Dogs in this group may be identical in temperament to the more aggressive dogs in Groups 5 and 6; however, Group 4 dogs have been influenced by training to obey their handlers' *down* command, even in the presence of strange dogs in their own territories. The dog in Group 4 knows that its owner is the boss. If you have trained your dog to be in Group 4 instead of Groups 5 or 6, you will be able to control its actions. You can add another dog to your pack without a great deal of difficulty.

Group 5

Just as with Group 4, Group 5 dogs will challenge strangers with stiff legs, growls, snarls, and raised hackles. The difference is that dogs in Group 5 are so intent on defending their territories from other dogs that they will not obey handlers' commands to desist. Group 5 dogs must be physically prevented from escalating their challenges into attacks. It will take many introductory sessions before a dog in Group 5 will accept another dog, particularly an adult one of the same sex, as a fellow pack member.

Group 6

Group 6 dogs are dangerous to other dogs. A dog in this group does not hesitate—the instant it sees another dog, even away from home, a Group 6 dog launches a murderous attack. No amount of yelling by the handler, no amount of jerking on a choke chain or swatting with the end of the leash deters a Group 6 dog from its intent to kill.

A Group 6 dog may even redirect its aggression toward its handler if it cannot reach its intended victim. At the least, it is likely to bite the leash that restrains it. If allowed, Group 6

Consider Your Resident Dog's Behavior

If you want another dog, by all means, get one. You need not allow the behavior of your resident dog or dogs to make your decision; however, consider the behavior of your resident dog when you decide how to introduce the newcomer. Use appropriate caution and patience, and you will be successful.

dogs will go into a frenzy of aggression until they are exhausted, with bloody lips from attacking the leash and anything else within reach.

Severe measures must be taken before Group 6 dogs are willing to accept a truce with other dogs; in some cases, a truce is impossible. Owners of medium and large dogs in Group 6 must face the fact that their dogs may never be loose safely in the presence of other dogs. Fortunately, very few dogs are really in Group 6; most of those that seem to be members of Group 6 are really in Groups 4 or 5—these dogs are putting up a good bluff.

Don't be fooled by a dog that leaps to the end of its leash and barks frantically when it sees another dog. Barkers, particularly those of small breeds, probably are overexcited members of Group 2 and, after a few moments, they will be ready to sniff noses and accept a new friend. Real members of Group 6 do not bark; they just attack.

Caution: If you have a dog that *really* is a member of Group 6, consider not even obtaining another dog. The risk and inconvenience may not be worth the reward.

Chapter Five

The Correct Equipment for Control

Ownership of more than just one dog can be easy, or it can be difficult. Occasionally, it can be impossible. The difference is in the amount of control that you, the owner, can maintain over the actions of each of your animals. If each of your dogs behaved exactly as you wanted it to, there would be no problems. If each behaved exactly as *it* wishes, they might kill one another.

Dogs—most dogs—respond to praise and scolding from their owners; however, many dogs' actions are so controlled by their instinctive and learned behavior as to make praise and scolding alone ineffective to prevent aggression toward other dogs. Many dogs must be physically restrained until they learn to accept a newcomer into their homes, and dogs soon learn when their owners are unable to physically control them.

The degree of physical restraint needed for each dog depends on these three variables: the disposition of the dog, the size of the dog, and the physical ability of its owner. Getting the job done with a minimum of difficulty requires using the correct equipment (see page 135 for addresses of sources for dog equipment).

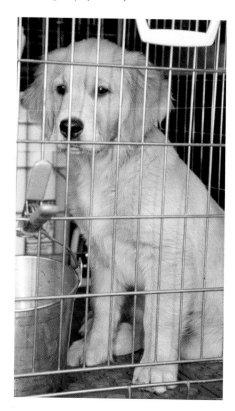

This little guy is comfortable in his safe place.

Dog Enclosures— the Safe Place

The most basic item in dog control is an enclosure in which the dog can be confined when the owner is not able to directly influence its actions. This enclosure is called a *safe place* because the confined dog is safe from harm and from causing harm. Every dog should have its own safe place whenever it enters a new environment. Once a dog has learned acceptable behavior, the use of its safe place may be discontinued except in unusual circumstances.

The most commonly used safe place is a housebreaking cage. To train a puppy to eliminate only outside the house, it should be confined to a cage at times when the owner cannot supervise its actions. The puppy's instinct to keep its bed clean discourages it from messing in the cage. It is released from its safe place at appropriate intervals. Each time it is released, the puppy is taken to the area chosen by its owner as the "bathroom" to urinate and defecate before it is allowed supervised freedom in the house.

The use in housebreaking is only one of the many advantages of every dog having a safe place. Confinement in its safe place prevents a dog from destroying household furnishings and harming or being harmed by other animals in the household. Each dog should have its own safe place in which it can be confined until its actions demonstrate that it no longer needs confinement.

The requirements of an appropriate safe place are simple:

- *The safe place must be escape-proof.* It must be made of sturdy material that the dog cannot destroy. It must have a top, or high sides that the dog cannot climb or jump. It must have a latch on its door that the dog cannot paw open.
- *A safe place should admit light.* No dog should be required to spend its time in darkness. It should be located in a dry and warm area where the dog can see household activity.
- *The safe place must be large enough for the dog.* The dog should be able to stand up and raise its head, turn around, and lie down in comfort. When building or buying a safe place, consider the size of the dog as an adult, not as a puppy. Dog enclosures are expensive to buy and troublesome to build, so make it large enough for the full-grown dog. Regard each dog's safe place as a permanent installation even though it might not often be used once the dog is trained.

Restraint Equipment—Collars and Leashes

Buckle-on Collars

Buckle-on dog collars are the first restraint used on puppies, and are the main restraint used on dogs that are easy to control. Buckle-on collars consist of a strap of leather or fabric (usually nylon) with a buckle on one end and holes for adjustment on the other. These collars have a D-ring for a leash sewn or riveted near the buckle. Buckled collars are obtainable in an infinite variety of sizes, weights, and design to suit every size of puppy and dog. Many of these collars can be lengthened as the puppy grows.

Buckle-on collars are the most mild of dog-restraint equipment. They are for use on puppies and toy and small breeds that are easy to restrain. Buckled collars can also be used on all dogs in Groups 1 and 2, dogs that have no intention of fighting with other dogs or of attacking other animals.

A newer development in canine haberdashery is a nylon buckled collar designed for flyball competition. This collar has a built-in handle that makes it easy for the handler to grab the dog by the collar. A collar of this sort can be useful for anyone who needs to restrain a dog without a leash.

"Choke" or "Slip" Collars

Both "choke" and "slip" mean the same thing. The term "choke" defines what these collars do: They close on a dog's neck with a choking action. "Slip collar" is a sugar-coated term for a choke collar, so named because it is slipped over the dog's head.

A choke collar consists of a chain or a fabric cord with a ring at each

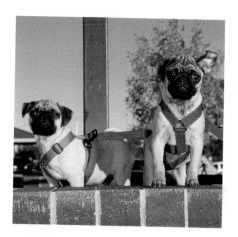

A harness on each is enough to control these little Pug puppies.

end. The collar is formed into a loop by passing the chain or cord through one of the rings. The loop is then slipped over the dog's head and around its neck. The dog is disciplined by tightening the loop with a pull on the leash attached to the free ring. The pressure of the choke collar on the dog's throat acts as an uncomfortable stimulus when the leash is tightened.

The approved method in obedience training of using a choke collar is for the handler to use sharp, short jerks with the leash to correct "wrong" responses by the dog, but, as with all correction equipment, choke collars have a great potential for misuse. Dogs have very muscular necks; medium and large dogs can easily ignore momentary tightening of the collar around their throats. The handler, frustrated by the dog's lack of response, may resort to using the choke collar too severely. The handler may place the collar just behind the dog's ears, jerk the leash with great force, or maintain pressure on

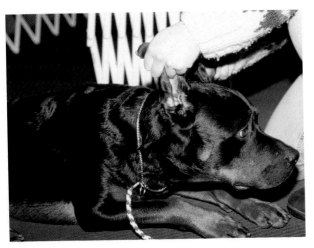

This Rottweiler is wearing a chain choke collar.

limited-choke collar is a useful tool on a dog with a relatively small head and thick neck such as a Greyhound or a Doberman Pinscher. When adjusted correctly, this collar is very mild in its action.

An advantage to the choke collar (chain, nylon, or limited-choke) is that it tightens when the leash is pulled. The wearer cannot back out of the collar as it might with a plain buckled collar.

Choke collars can be of use on small dogs in Groups 3, 4, and 5, and on medium and large dogs in Group 3 and 4. A medium or large dog in Groups 5 or 6 will need stronger measures.

If you decide to use a choke collar on any of your dogs, be determined to use it properly.

• Resolve to never use the collar to "strangle" your dog. Give only short corrections, followed by instant releases.

• Remember that a thick chain choke collar is much more humane than a thin nylon choke. If you cannot control your dog unless the choke is fitted tightly behind your dog's ears, you should use another device.

• Be sure the collar fits the dog. When the collar is pulled tight, there should be no more than 2 to 3 inches (5–7.6 cm) of slack in the chain or cord. A properly fitted collar will loosen by its own weight the instant leash pressure is released.

• Thick chains apply pressure to a larger area on dogs' throats than do thin ones, so are less severe. Select

the leash until the dog's windpipe is closed. Dogs have had their hyoid bones (small bones in the base of the tongue) crushed, and have even been choked into insensibility or death by improper use of the choke collar. This is why some knowledge-able dog trainers call these devices "strangle collars."

Choke collars made of chain are more humane than those made of nylon. Nylon chokes, particularly those of thin cord, do not fall open as readily as do chains when leash pressure is released. The sound made by a chain collar when it is tightened warns the dog that a correction is imminent, a factor not present with the use of a nylon cord choker.

A useful variation of the nylon choke is the limited-choke collar, sometimes called a "greyhound collar" or a "martingale collar." These are adjustable, made of nylon in various widths, and feature a loop-and-ring device that can tighten the collar to only a limited extent. The

the collar of the correct length with the thickest links possible.

- Small dogs with choke collars need special consideration. Never jerk a leash attached to a choke collar on a small dog with enough force to yank the dog off the ground. You may injure it severely.

Dog Halters or Headcollars: A Humane Choice

There are many dogs, particularly large, aggressive types, which cannot be influenced by a choke collar *used correctly*. If you have one of these, do not use the collar incorrectly; obtain a better training tool.

Cattle and horses are controlled by rope or leather halters fitted around the animals' heads. By attaching the leads close to the end of the jaws, handlers are able to control animals that far exceed them in strength and weight. Similar devices are now manufactured for dog control.

Dog headcollars operate on the principle that *when you control the head, you control the whole dog.* Headcollars afford instant and nearly effortless control of even large and unruly dogs. In virtually every instance, headcollars are the most effective and the most humane form of restraint devices.

Headcollars fit around the dog's muzzle, and fasten behind its ears. The leash is attached to a ring below the dog's jaw. The strap around the muzzle tightens when the leash is pulled, which acts to close the dog's mouth. Headcollars do not restrict a dog's breathing, nor do they prevent

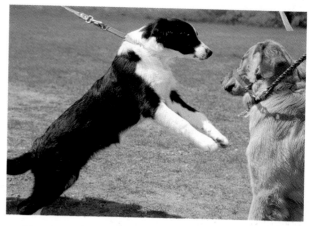

a dog from opening its mouth to pant. These devices are excellent for use on dogs in Groups 4, 5, and 6. Owners of medium and large dogs in Groups 2 and 3 will also enjoy the extra control afforded by headcollars.

Dog headcollars are made of nylon, come in many sizes, and are lightweight, durable, and washable. They have only a few drawbacks:

- Dogs must become used to the feel of the headcollars around their muzzles before they will ignore them. Dogs that are not accustomed to headcollars will try to remove them with their claws. Most dogs learn to tolerate the headcollar in only a lesson or two.
- It is important to select the correct size of headcollar for each dog. The headcollar must be fitted correctly and securely so that the dog cannot pull out of it.
- Headcollars cannot be left on unattended dogs, indoors or outdoors. Headcollars on unattended dogs may become caught on objects and strangle the wearers.

In spite of its limited-choke nylon collar, the Border Collie is willing to jump on the Golden Retriever.

- Owners may have to struggle to get the headcollars on their dogs the first several times they are used. Eventually, dogs can be trained to not resist when the headcollars are applied.
- Headcollars are not allowed in show rings or in field trials. Neither are pinch collars, electronic collars, nor any devices other than buckled collars or choke collars. A dog intended for exhibition may be trained at home using a headcollar, but it must also learn to obey wearing only equipment approved for the competition.

Pinch, Spike, Prong, or Tack Collars

All the terms—pinch, spike, prong, and tack—mean the same thing: a collar that has some sort of projections on the inside surface. When the collar is tightened, the projections contact the dog's neck. Depending on the sharpness of the projections and the degree to which the collar is tightened, the dog feels anything from a mild pinching sensation to severe pain. Few dogs will ignore a pinch collar. These devices also have a great potential for abuse.

Pinch collars are sized for small, medium, and large dogs, and can be purchased in two forms. The more common type is made of stout wire links, each link with two short wire projections that contact the dog's neck. The links are fitted together to form the collar. The links at each end are passed through a chain loop to which the leash is attached. When the leash is pulled, the chain loop tightens the collar.

Pinch collars are adjusted to size by adding or removing links. A pinch collar should be adjusted so that the prongs just contact the dog's neck. If the collar is too loose, its effect will be lost unless the handler yanks the leash with excessive force. Properly adjusted, a pinch collar is too small to be slipped over the dog's head. The collar must be unfastened and buckled around the dog's neck each time it is put on or removed.

Metal-link pinch collars are now available with rubber-tipped, "humane" prongs. The rubber tips prevent the collar from scratching the dog's skin and somewhat soften the effect of the collar. After months of use, these rubber tips tend to fall off.

Another type of pinch collar resembles a flat leather choke collar through which short blunt tacks have been sewn. The collar is adjustable by means of a buckle end. These collars are correctly termed "tack" collars or "force collars." They are slightly less difficult to fit and use than are the all-metal pinch collars, but the tacks may be sharper, thus increasing the potential for abuse. These collars can be made more humane by blunting the tacks with a file.

Although it may look brutal, the pinch collar is a more humane alternate than is the incorrect use of the common choke collar. The pinch collar cannot strangle or choke a dog. When the leash is tightened, the pinch collar pricks the dog's neck with several points. The force applied, the sharpness of the points, the thickness of the dog's coat, and the sensitivity of the animal are factors that determine how dogs respond to corrections given with pinch collars.

Pinch collars are of use on dogs in Groups 5 and 6. If you decide to use one of these, use it properly:

- Adjust the collar correctly. The prongs should barely touch the dog's skin. If these collars are too loose, it takes a violent yank of the leash to deliver a correction.
- Never use more force than is absolutely necessary to get your dog's attention.
- Never use a pinch collar that is sharp enough to pierce skin. It is inexcusable to cause actual wounds in the skin of your dog's neck.
- Never use a pinch collar with a continuous pull on the leash. Even blunt points can damage skin when applied with constant pressure.
- In almost all instances in which a pinch collar is necessary, a better and more humane choice is the dog headcollar.

Shock Collars

Of all the available dog-control equipment, none has as much potential for abuse as does the electric shock collar.

Shock collars consist of two parts:
1. a buckle-type receiver collar with two terminals (prongs) that contact the dog's skin, and

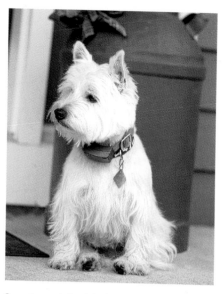

Even small dogs can wear electronic fence collars.

2. a hand-held, battery-powered transmitter that delivers an electric shock to the wearer when the operator presses a button. These collars have many variations; most are adjustable to deliver progressively stronger shocks to the dog.

The use of a shock collar to prevent fighting among dogs can never be recommended for these reasons:
1. The shocked dog may think that the other dog is causing the shock. In some cases, notably dogs in Group 6, the shocked dog may retaliate by attacking more fiercely or may redirect its aggression toward the handler.
2. Dogs are very quick to realize that they cannot be shocked when they are not wearing the shock collar, and that they cannot be shocked when the handler with the transmitter is not present.

29

Dogs inhibited from fighting by use of a shock collar will not be inhibited in the absence of their handlers.

3. Electronic collars of every sort are prohibited on show and field-trial grounds; therefore, the dog trained with an electronic device may be out of control when the device is removed.

4. Shock collars are expensive and fragile; they need frequent repair and battery replacement. Save your money.

Muzzles

A dog muzzle is intended to prevent the dog that is wearing one from being able to bite. Dog muzzles are of several types:

The basket muzzle. This consists of a cagelike basket, usually made of wire, plastic, woven leather strips, or a combination of materials. The muzzle is held in place over the dog's nose and mouth by leather or fabric straps that fasten behind the dog's ears. A dog wearing a basket muzzle can open its mouth to pant, but cannot get its teeth into anything that cannot pass through the openings in the basket. A dog wearing a wire basket muzzle can injure its

Be Careful!

Never use any type of muzzle to replace caution. Never even *think* about allowing two muzzled dogs to "fight it out." One or both muzzles will become dislodged; one or both dogs will be seriously injured.

handler and dislodge the basket when it struggles or tries to attack another dog. There are many better muzzles than the basket variety.

The leather strap muzzle. These muzzles are constructed of straps designed to hold a dog's mouth closed so that it cannot bite. To be effective, they must be very tight; however, they do not stay tight because leather stretches. A dog with a loose muzzle can bite quite effectively. The use of a leather strap muzzle is not recommended. It may give handlers a false sense of security.

The nylon-strap muzzle. Nylon is a much more durable substance from which to construct control equipment than is leather. Many nylon-strap muzzles have Velcro adjustments. When applied tight enough to be effective, these muzzles are hardly humane. They should not be used on a dog for more than a few minutes at a time.

The nylon cone muzzle. If you must use a muzzle, use a nylon cone. These are the most humane, the most effective, the lightest in weight, and the least expensive of all types of muzzles. The cone muzzle fits snugly over the dog's mouth; the end of the cone is open so that the nose is not covered and the dog can breathe. Cone muzzles come in many sizes, including those for short-faced breeds. They must be fitted carefully. If the muzzle is too large for the dog, it will be able to bite while wearing it. A nice variation of the nylon cone muzzle is the one with a tab and ring for a leash sewn onto the bottom of the cone. This allows the device to act as a halter and muzzle combined.

Leashes and Chains

Never leave a dog tied with a leather or nylon leash. Almost all dogs will escape by biting through leather, fabric, or rope. *Never* lead a dog by a chain. When it pulls, it will damage your hands. You may even need gloves when leading a very strong dog on a leather or fabric leash.

The important feature of a leash is that it must be strong enough to hold the dog to which it is attached. Big dogs need thick, wide leashes;

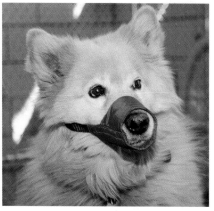

This mixed breed models a humane nylon cone muzzle.

small dogs can be restrained by very thin leashes. Nylon is the strongest material for leashes, and also the most durable. Leather and cotton

The Most Common Startle Devices Are:

1. An object that makes noise when thrown toward a dog, such as a piece of chain or a soda can containing pebbles or a few pennies. It is not necessary to hit the dog with the noisemaker to achieve the startle effect, only to hit the ground near the dog.

2. An object that makes noise at the touch of a button. A number of hand-held noisemakers are available from pet supply companies. Some of these produce sound above humans' range of hearing (ultrasound); some produce loud noise that humans as well as dogs can hear ("bark-breakers" intended to startle dogs enough to inhibit their barking). Boat stores sell foghorn-type canisters intended to be used to signal

other ships. After a number of applications, however, dogs tend to become used to the noises and these devices may lose their effectiveness.

3. A device to spray water on the dog. Turning a garden hose on fighting dogs is the classic example. A less severe alternate is a water pistol directed at the aggressor. A squirt from a compressed air canister, which also makes a hissing noise, is more appropriate indoors. These canisters are used to blow dust off delicate electronic equipment and are available at computer and electronics stores. *Do not* use the ones that contain chemicals for cleaning electronic equipment.

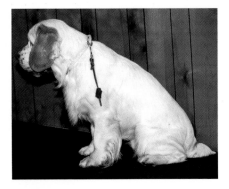

The Clumber Spaniel wears a short leash for its owner to grab.

web leashes are satisfactory if they are inspected regularly for wear.

Leash snaps should be sturdy; brass snaps outlast steel ones. Snaps with hinged tongues may be stronger than bolt snaps, but both can break. Some very inexpensive leashes have flimsy snaps that break easily; cheap leashes do not last long; they are not a good way to save money.

Dog tie-out chains are usually made of twisted wire figure-eight links of various weights for large, medium, or small dogs. The difference in the price of dog chains depends on their length, weight, and quality of hard-ware. Inexpensive chains will have weak snaps and swivels that will function adequately for small dogs but will be pulled apart by larger ones.

"Startle" Devices

A "startle" device is an object intended to frighten or distract a dog from committing an undesirable action. The "startle" should take place the instant the handler recognizes that the dog is about to act inappropriately. For example, a puppy should be startled the instant it starts to squat on the rug. The startle inhibits the action, so the puppy can be taken to the appropriate location to eliminate. When introducing two dogs, the aggressor can be startled the instant it growls which acts to take its attention away from the other animal.

Dogs in Groups 1, 2, and 3 usually respond well to startle devices; members of Groups 4, 5, and 6 will not be deterred from aggression. Don't rely on startling to inhibit dogs in these groups.

Obtain the Correct Equipment before You Need It

Size of Dog	Suggested Collar
Small dogs in Groups 1, 2, and 3	Plain buckled collar of leather or nylon
Small dogs in Groups 4, 5, and 6	Headcollar or chain choke collar
Medium dogs in Groups 1 and 2	Plain collar or choke chain
Medium dogs in Groups 3, 4, and 5	Headcollar or chain choke collar
Medium dogs in Group 6	Headcollar or pinch collar
Large dogs in Groups 1 and 2	Headcollar or chain choke
Large dogs in Groups 3, 4, and 5	Headcollar or pinch collar
Large dogs in Group 6	Headcollar, pinch collar, or muzzle/halter combo

Chapter Six

The Basic Commands

Dogs can be trained to obey astonishingly complex commands. Dogs herd livestock, obeying whistle and hand signals. They guide the blind through city traffic. They perform unbelievable circus tricks. They act in movies in which they outshine the human actors. They perform exercises of surprising intricacy in obedience and agility trials. Every one of these talented dogs started their education in the same way—they learned to obey the basic commands.

When Do Dogs Disobey?

Dogs disobey *only* when they are insufficiently trained. Your dog is not spiteful nor resentful when it does not obey a command. Your dog is ignorant. Oh, yes, your dog might disobey a command that you know it understands. It understands the command but is not trained well enough to always obey even when it would rather do something else.

It is the trainer, not the dog, who is at fault if a dog fails to obey a command *every time*. The dog that appears to be stupid, stubborn, or willful needs a more patient and determined trainer.

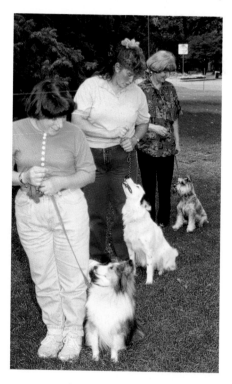

The handler is more than half of the team.

Which Commands Are Essential?

To be in complete control of your dog's actions, you do not need to train it to run through mazes, to track fugitives, or to obey hand signals. By training only a few basic commands, you can govern your dog's behavior in the most difficult of situations.

The *sit* command is not essential, but is trained first because it is so easy for the trainer to teach and the dog to understand. It gives both handler and dog a quick and successful start in the training process.

The two commands that are absolutely essential for your dog to obey are *come* and *down (down-stay)*. A dog that always obeys these two commands can be called away from potential dogfights. It can be called back from chasing other animals. It can be prevented from acting hostile or predatory toward other animals. By enforcing these two commands, handlers are able to control their dogs' aggressive actions in every circumstance.

If You Compete with Your Dog

Dogs trained for obedience or agility trials, dog shows, or field trials are expected to follow different standards of performance than are dogs that are not competitors. It is a major fault in the obedience ring if a dog sits during the *down-stay* exercise. At home, it makes absolutely no difference whether the dog is sitting or lying down, as long as it remains where it was commanded to stay. In the obedience ring, the *come* command indicates that the dog is to come to a sitting position directly in front of the handler. Hunting dogs are usually taught to come to the *heel* position next to the handler's left leg. A dog must obey with precision in obedience trials; at home and in the hunting field, perfect precision is not important. It is obeying the basic action that is important.

Decide if you will enter your dog in competitions. Study a current copy of the rule book for your event and train your dog to the level of accuracy the competition requires. If you have no competitive ambition for your dog, you need only to train it to obey the basic elements of the action. You need not worry about such details as a crooked *sit*.

You can always change your mind. When you take your dog to obedience classes, you might be inspired to enter your dog in obedience trials. If so, you can improve the accuracy of the commands it already knows, and you can teach your dog a new command for any exercise it performs in a nonregulation manner. If you trained your dog to come to the *heel* position next to your left leg, you can teach it another command (*front*) to come to the sitting position directly in front of you as is required in the obedience ring.

Shorten Your Vocabulary of Commands

Your dog must learn a new language: yours. The fewer words in your dog's dictionary, the faster the dog will be able to understand you; therefore, analyze every command and eliminate those that are unnecessary.

- *Sit!* means *"Sit and stay there."* In every instance in which your dog is instructed to sit, *stay* is also implied. Why confuse your dog with an extra word? To a dog, *Sit!* always means *"Sit there until your handler tells you to do something else."*
- *Down!* means *"Lie down and stay there."* Just as with *sit,* the *stay* is a redundant command. Your dog does not need to learn that extra word.
- *Come!* means *"Go to a sitting position directly in front of, close to, and facing your handler."* A dog that is not entered in obedience competitions need not come and sit in front of its handler as long as it comes close enough for the handler to touch it. The dog can be trained to come to the *heel* position if the handler prefers.
- *"Okay"* is the universal release command. You can use another word if you wish. *"Okay"* means that the dog is free to do whatever it desires. Use this command only at the conclusion of each exercise. If you do not intend for the dog to be released from your control, do not say *"Okay";* lead it or direct it to its next exercise.

Training with the Correct Leash and Collar

For these simple obedience exercises, obtain a 6-foot (1.8 m) leash of a thickness appropriate to the size of your dog. The leash can be made of leather, cloth, or nylon, but not chain.

Headcollars

Your choice of collar depends on the size and disposition of your dog. For most dogs that weigh over 30 pounds (13.6 kg), a headcollar is the best option (see page 27). No dog wearing a headcollar can effectively resist its handler's control, yet the headcollar causes the dog no pain and can produce no injury to the dog's throat.

Headcollars are not allowed in obedience or agility competitions, nor in field trials. If you intend to compete with your dog, first train with a headcollar. When the dog will obey off leash while wearing the headcollar, it will obey off leash without it. Once the dog is obedient, have it wear both the headcollar and a regular collar for several training sessions. Snap the leash onto the regular collar but try to keep the leash slack. Eventually you will be able to remove the headcollar.

If your dog will not obey with the leash on its regular collar, it simply has not been trained thoroughly. Practice, practice, practice with the leash and headcollar until it will obey without them.

Many dogs smaller than 30 pounds (13.6 kg) may be trained effectively with a simple buckled collar. Use a headcollar even on a small dog if your dog ignores your leash corrections or tries to drag you around. If you decide to use a choke collar, resolve to use it correctly. Do not use a choke collar as an instrument of strangulation.

Training Tips

Praise and Encouragement

"Good boy" (or "girl") should be a major part of every dog's vocabulary. Every correct response should earn the dog enthusiastic praise and a loving pat. Even if your dog seems relatively unresponsive to your praise, it will recognize when its actions meet with your approval.

On the other hand, praise should never be given in an overly enthusiastic way. Praise should never be an excuse to allow your dog to jump around out of control, even for a minute. Praise should never be used as a release command. Following a correct response to a command, the proper way to praise your dog is to lean over, give it a couple of pats on the shoulder, chest, or flank, and tell it, "Good Boy" (or "Girl") in a happy tone of voice. While being praised, the dog should remain in the indicated position, alert and ready to receive another command. If your dog gets too excited by praise, use praise only after you have given the release command, and do not praise with too much enthusiasm. Praise is an acknowledgment that the dog is doing the proper thing; it is not an excuse to go wild.

Correction in its mildest form is the absence of praise. Your dog earns no praise when it does not obey. The appropriate verbal correction for a dog that fails to obey a command is to repeat the command while simultaneously enforcing it. There is no reason to startle or confuse the dog by shouting "Bad Dog." Here is the correct sequence:

1. You command *"Sit,"* the dog sits, you lean over, pat it, and say "Good Dog."
2. If the dog starts to get up before you have released it, you repeat the *sit* command while you push it back into the sitting position.
3. If necessary, you do this dozens of times. Eventually the dog gets the idea; it stays in the sitting position until you say *"Okay."*

Food Rewards

Make training a pleasant experience for your dog. Although you will train with a combination of the inductive (persuasion) and compulsive (force) methods, make training fun. The dog that receives food rewards early in its training will be the dog that regards all training with enthusiasm.

Of course, eventually, your dog must obey even when you do not have a pocket full of goodies. For instance, rewarding your dog with food is prohibited in the obedience ring. As your dog's education progresses, you can phase out food rewards by offering them less often, then very infrequently, then never.

Food as a reward should be something different and much more desirable to your dog than its regular diet. Many trainers use small pieces of cheese or tiny cubes of boiled liver as rewards. These have to be prepared ahead of time, often stick together, and spoil when you forget them and leave them in your pocket. Successful items to use as food rewards are pieces of semimoist cat treats. Cat treats are available in grocery stores, come in handy little containers, and in a variety of flavors. Most dogs love them. These little pieces of food will pick up lint in your pocket (which does not affect their desirability to your dog) but are not as messy as cheese or liver.

Teach Your Dog to Learn

Dogs and all other animals (including humans) must learn how to learn. A puppy or a dog that has had little human contact does not know that a "noise" made by a person can have a specific meaning and should elicit a specific response. Dogs learn this when they learn to associate a noise with an action carried out by a human.

The first noise a dog learns is the sound of its own name. For example: Your new puppy is Buster, but you can say "Buster, Buster,

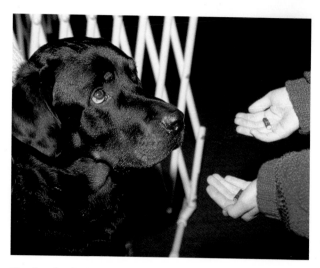

Buster," all day and the puppy will ignore you, because he does not know that the noise applies to him in any way. If you say "Buster" whenever you approach the pup, and "Good Buster" (with enthusiasm) whenever you pat him or offer him food, Buster will learn that the spoken word, "Buster" precedes pleasant interaction with you. He will give you his attention and probably come to you whenever you say "Buster." He will have learned that a sound can have meaning; in other words, Buster will have learned his name.

Once a puppy learns that a specific sound (its name) has a specific meaning ("*Look at me*"), it will be ready to learn the meaning of other spoken words.

Train Where There Are No Distractions

The worst place in the world to teach your dog a new command is in an obedience class. The command is

Teach your dog to wait for its treat.

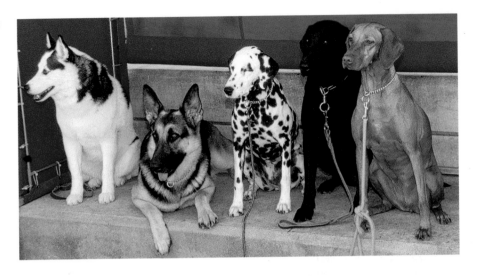

Any breed can learn to obey.

unfamiliar to the dog and the environment is unfamiliar to the dog. Worst of all, there are other dogs present to occupy your dog's attention. With all these distractions, how can you expect your dog to learn?

Start to teach every new command in a familiar environment in which no other animals are present. If people are watching, ask them to sit quietly and not disturb the lesson. Only after your dog has learned the meaning of the new command should you ask it to obey in novel situations and in the presence of other animals.

The best obedience instructors schedule the first class of each novice obedience course to be for owners without their dogs. The instructors bring their own dogs or one or two volunteers' dogs to demonstrate correct training technique. The instructors show owners how to start teaching the commands

at home, so that the dog can begin to learn them in a familiar environment.

Members of obedience training classes are encouraged to give their dogs at least one short lesson at home every day. Any dog that has received six or more lessons of a simple exercise will certainly recognize the command word, even if it does not obey it perfectly. The dog will then be prepared to obey the command while in the presence of other dogs and in a confusing environment

At the conclusion of each novice obedience class, the best instructors demonstrate the new exercise for the following week, to allow owners to familiarize their dogs with each new exercise at home. This becomes less important after three or four weeks of classes, once the dogs have become accustomed to the distractions and pay better attention to their handlers.

Make Training Fun

When you make training fun, when you offer food rewards, when you use plenty of praise and rarely use punishment, your dog will want to obey you. It is easy to train a dog to obey—as long as it wants to. It will want to obey until a squirrel dashes past or it gets a whiff of the neighbor's dog; then it might run off and ignore your commands. Many dogs are perfect on leash, but out of control when the leash is removed.

A great deal of effort and ingenuity has been expended in trying to convince dogs that they were still under restraint when their leashes were removed. Trainers have attached long thin cords (even very strong fishing line) to dogs' collars, thinking that the dogs will not notice a very lightweight line. When the dogs disobey, the trainers have tried to "surprise" them with the fact that they are still on leash. These trainers soon realize that dogs are not that stupid; they can see and feel any rope strong enough to hold them. When the rope is gone, so is the obedience.

Trainers cannot run after a dog to punish it for disobedience. Almost any dog can run faster than almost any person; a dog that expects punishment is not willing to allow itself to be caught.

Dog training has recently entered the electronic age. Collars have been developed that allow handlers to give dogs an electric shock at distances of up to a mile. These devices have some value, but they have serious drawbacks. They are quite expensive and they often malfunction. Used incorrectly, a collar that delivers an electric shock to a dog obviously constitutes cruelty.

As with the light rope, dogs can tell if they are wearing an electronic collar. Electronic collars are heavy and contain batteries that a dog can detect by the odor. Dogs trained electronically must be persuaded to obey without the shock collars if they are to be entered in competitions. Electronic shock collars and anything resembling them are prohibited in all dog shows and trials.

Train Your Dog On Leash to Obey Off Leash

If neither long ropes nor electronic collars are humane and successful methods to train a dog to obey off leash, what is? It's very simple: Train your dog *on leash* to obey *off leash.* Practice, practice, practice until your dog is mentally so conditioned that it cannot disobey your commands, even in the presence of severe temptation.

Trainers whose dogs refuse to obey off leash are trainers who have made a basic mistake—they took off the leash too soon. Trainers are always tempted to see if their dogs will perform off leash. Every dog realizes immediately when it is not wearing a leash. The first time a dog makes a mistake off leash and the trainer is unable to correct it, the dog begins to learn that the leash is the trainer's source of authority. When the dog has disobeyed a few times without being corrected, it has learned this lesson: *No leash, no authority!*

Take the leash off your dog only when it has performed faultlessly for weeks on a slack leash. Remove the leash when the necessity for giving your dog a leash correction is only a memory. Then, and only then, try off-leash training at home and with a piece of food in your hand. Try off-leash training at obedience class only when your dog is absolutely perfect at home. At the first sign of disobedience, put the leash right back on.

Some dogs require an enormous amount of training before they will consistently obey off leash. Older dogs that have had years of experience in ignoring their owners' instructions may take months of daily lessons before they can be depended upon to come or heel off leash. It will only happen if you practice, practice, practice.

Books Can Help You Train

Public libraries and bookstores are full of volumes that tell you how to train your dog. The bibliography at the end of this book contains the titles of several good ones. Authors each express their individual attitudes toward discipline, but you will see that the methods of training each command are very similar in nearly all the books. Go to the library and examine the selection. Pick out one or two that seem to give you the most understandable instructions, check them out, and read them thoroughly. You might want to buy the one you like best to keep at home for reference.

It is fun and rewarding to train your dog to perform the many complicated exercises explained in these books, but to keep control of your dog in the presence of other animals, you need teach only the basic commands.

Sit

Start your training with the *sit* command because it is the easiest exercise a dog can learn. Dogs (except those of the Greyhound type) spend much of their time in the sitting position. You do not have to teach your dog *sit*; you only have to teach it to sit when you give the command.

First Lesson

1. Use the inductive method to teach your dog the meaning of *sit*—use a food reward. Start with the dog on leash, so it cannot go far from you. Training *sit* on leash also serves to associate the leash with food rewards in the dog's mind.

2. Select your own word that will mean *release from control* to your dog. "*Okay*" is used most often, but you can use any word you choose. Use this word only to mean release from your control; do not use the word as praise. For example, do not release your dog

by saying "Good Dog" unless you are never going to say "Good Dog" when giving praise.

3. Allow the dog to see the food in your hand, but do not allow it to jump on you to try to reach it. If it does, step back to prevent the dog's front paws from contacting your legs.

4. Hold the food right over the dog's head, so that it will look up to keep the treat in view. As it looks up, it will naturally sit. The instant it sits, say: *"Sit!"* and give it the food. Then say *"Okay"* (or your own release command) and allow it to rise. Pet and praise your dog if you want to, but in this exercise, the food is the main reward.

It will take very few repetitions before your dog will automatically sit as it sees your hand raised above its head. Most dogs learn this with only a half-dozen pieces of cat treats. The dog will learn this sequence: First, command *"Sit!"* Second, raise your hand with a treat. Third, the dog sits in anticipation of the treat. Fourth, the dog receives the treat. Fifth, give the release command, *"Okay."*

Second Lesson

At the second lesson—yes, your dog will learn that much in one lesson—try to eliminate the second step in the sequence. Have a treat in your hand but do not show it to the dog. Say *"Sit!"* without raising your hand. If the dog sits, give it the treat immediately. If it does not, repeat *"Sit"* as you raise your hand, wait until it sits, then give it the treat.

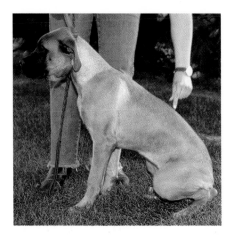

Practice this until your dog will nearly always sit on command without seeing your hand raised. Never forget to give the release command at the end of each exercise.

Third Lesson

At the third lesson, begin to phase out the food reward. Give the dog a treat only every third or fourth time it obeys the *sit* command. Always vary the pattern—give two treats in a row, then none for three commands. Or give a treat every other time. The dog should always anticipate a treat but never know when it is going to get one. At this stage in training, do not eliminate food rewards entirely.

Fourth Lesson

During the fourth lesson it is time to teach your dog that it must obey the *sit* command, even if it is doing something more interesting. This will be hard to do, because *sit* is so easy and the food reward has made compliance so pleasant that your dog ordinarily will never fail to

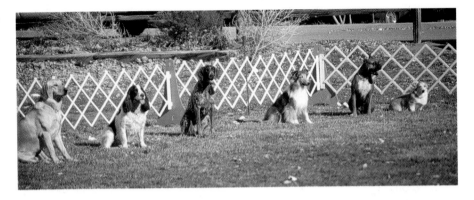

Dogs performing a long sit in obedience class.

obey. Command *"Sit"* at the door when the dog is eager to go outside. Practice in a different location where there are fascinating new smells. If your dog does not immediately sit on command, there is nothing wrong with adding a little compulsion to your training: Push it into the *sit* position while repeating the command *"Sit!"* Insist on instant obedience. Offer food rewards only five or six times in the entire lesson.

Fifth Lesson

Remember, *sit* actually means *sit-stay*. At the fifth lesson, it is time to enforce the *stay* portion of the command.

Practice until your dog will sit near you for a full 30 seconds, waiting for the release command. If your dog gets up without hearing your release command, push it back into the sitting position while you repeat *"sit."*

Then command *"Sit"* and take a single step away from the dog. Be careful not to tighten the leash. If the dog starts to get up, step back toward the dog, say *"Sit"* and push it back into position. When it will stay for 30 seconds with you one step away, practice this for two steps, three steps, eventually a dozen steps, insisting that the dog stay in the sitting position at all times. When you can leave your dog for three or four steps, drop the leash but keep it attached to the dog. Grab the leash when you have to make a correction.

If the dog gets up when you tell it to sit, take it back to the exact spot it left. Your goal is to have the dog remain sitting on the spot when you turn and walk away, and stay on the spot until you come back and give it the release command.

Never give the release command at a distance from the dog and never offer food when the dog is expected to stay. The sight (or even the anticipation) of a food reward will encourage the dog to come to you to get its treat. For the same reason, do not use the dog's name as part of a verbal correction. If the dog starts to get up when it is supposed to be sitting, say *"Sit!"* in a firm voice, and push it back into position. Do not say *"Buster, sit,"* because the sound of its name will encourage Buster to come to you. When the dog disobeys, there is no need to get angry or to yank your dog around. Be firm and patient, never abusive.

Note. Do not expect your dog to behave as well in obedience class as it does at home. It will take a few lessons in the presence of the other dogs before your dog learns that the rules are the same in class.

Down

"Down!" This command takes all the fun out of a dog's life. A dog obeying *"Down!"* cannot run into the road. It cannot beg for food. It cannot chase rabbits or attack the meter reader. Most important, a dog obeying the *down* command cannot get into a fight with another dog. Obedience to the *down* command is absolutely essential to control the behavior of a dog that might act aggressively toward other animals.

Dogs resist being placed in the *down* position; they find the position to be very repressive. A dog forced to lie in one place is removed from interaction with everything in its environment. A dog in the *down* position feels vulnerable to every human and animal that towers over it. *Down* is trained early in your dog's education for that very reason—to teach the dog that it must yield to your authority and do something it dislikes. The dog well-trained

in *down* will be quick to obey other commands, even when it would rather not.

The *down* command is not easy to teach. It is nearly impossible to teach to most dogs by the inductive method alone. Since dogs do not like to obey the command, there is almost nothing that will induce them to do so. Trainers have tried kneeling and holding a piece of food on the ground in front of a sitting dog. When the dog reaches for the food, these trainers slide the food forward, expecting that the dog will lie down while following the food with its nose, but this method only teaches the dog to grab food off the ground, not to lie down. To be successful, the *down* command must be taught by compelling, not inducing, the dog to obey.

Food Rewards

Use food rewards when teaching the *down* position, even though compulsion is required to get the dog in position. Reward your dog when it is in the *down* position with a treat on the ground between its front legs. Never offer a reward above the ground when you are training *down*. If you do, your dog will be encouraged to sit up to reach the treat.

Pulling Up on the Leash

Ignore the advice given in some books to place the leash under your instep and pull upward to force the dog's neck toward the ground. Most dogs will not understand this restraint and will struggle against it.

"Heel" can be on either side of the handler.

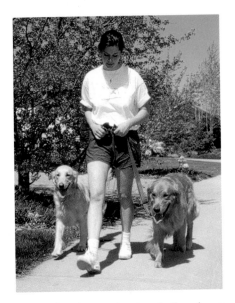

When the dog understands the *down* command, this procedure can be used to enforce the command if you wish.

Training Technique

The easiest way to train *down* is to give the command to a sitting dog while pulling its front legs forward. Kneel on the ground if you cannot accomplish this while you are standing. If the dog struggles to get its legs free, use one hand to pull its legs forward and the other hand to press its shoulders toward the ground. Hold the dog in position if you must, to prevent it from rising until you say *"Okay."* Here is the sequence:

1. Command *"Down"* while you place the dog in position by using your hands on its front legs and shoulders.
2. Quickly offer the treat on the ground between its front paws. If the dog struggles to rise, hold it down while you give it the treat. Soon it will stay in the correct position in anticipation of its reward.
3. Give the release command and allow the dog to rise.

You must do whatever necessary to get the dog into the *down* position, but try to accomplish this gently. Never grab the dog's front legs in one hand and its back legs in the other and slam it onto its side. Not only is this very frightening to a dog, but the normal *down* position for the dog is not on its side.

Remember, the verbal correction when your dog starts to get up is *"Down!"* not *"Buster, down!"* The sound of a dog's name will encourage it to get up to come to you. Do not forget the release command, *"Okay,"* every time you allow your dog to rise.

The *stay* portion of the *down* command is one of the most useful things you will ever teach your dog. Teach this just as you did the *stay* portion of the *sit* command: one step at a time. Be prepared to take a lot of time and patience until your dog will stay in place until you release it.

Come

You started to train your dog to obey the *come* command the first day you owned it: *"Buster, come!"* when you fed it, when you took it outdoors, whenever you and Buster were going to go somewhere together. Buster has already learned *sit (sit-stay)* when you walk away. Now you are ready to start Buster's "formal" training in *come*.

If you intend to compete in obedience trials with Buster, you should train him to come to a sitting position right in front of you. If Buster will be a field trial dog, you probably want him to come to the *heel* position next to your left leg. If Buster is not going to be a competitor, you may choose your own location for *come*, but you must be consistent; *"Buster, come"* must always mean the same thing.

First Lesson

For the first lesson, you will need a whole pocketful of cat treats. Take your dog, on leash, out in the yard or some other familiar place. Wait until its attention is not on you, then command *"Buster, come!"* as you run backward, holding out a treat. At the sound of his name, Buster looks at you. At the sight of the treat, he comes to get it. Repeat the command in an enthusiastic tone of voice as often as necessary to keep Buster coming toward you. When the dog sees the treat, you will not need to jerk on the leash. When he gets to you, guide him into the correct position, command *"Buster, sit,"* and give him the treat. Then give your release command.

Buster will probably stay close to you, hoping for more treats. Even if he is right at your feet, repeat the

Now You Are in Control!

When you taught your dog not to resist the submissive position, your dog learned to recognize you as its leader.

When you taught your dog the commands *down* and *come*, your dog learned to obey your wishes. Because you have been patient and persistent, your dog obeys every time.

Now you can control your dog's actions in all situations. You can insist that your dog live peacefully in a multiple-pet society.

exercise several times. Run backward and offer a treat while you encourage *"Buster, come!"* Practice the *sit* and *down* commands in between the *come* command.

Second Lesson

At the second lesson in *come*, ask Buster to come from the *sit* position. Leave him in *sit*. Back up to the end of the leash. Give the command *"Come"* as you run backward, drawing the dog toward you. After a few steps, stop, have Buster sit, and reward him with food.

If you ask your dog to come from the *sit* position too often, he will soon fail to stay in the *sit* position at all. Practice *come* only every seventh or eighth time; leave Buster in the *sit* position and walk around him (even out of his sight) without allowing him to come before you give the release command.

Chapter Seven

Acquiring Another Adult Dog

R over has been a member of your family for ten years. Now he is beginning to show his age—is it time to think about adding another dog?

"Let's get married! We'll live happily ever after." But will your dogs get along as happily as you do, or will they be constantly at each other's throats? Will your dogs be a source of friction in your new union? Is it fair to one partner to have to give up a dog just because the dogs do not get along?

There's a dog *exactly* like Queenie at the city kennels. If someone doesn't buy her, she will be destroyed. Will Queenie fight with her, or would she like a companion?

Mary has so much fun with Brandy in obedience trials; now Johnny wants a dog of his own to train. How can you deny one child the enjoyment you allow the other? But will Brandy allow another dog to enter his domain?

When you add another dog to your life, your family becomes one of the more than ten million multiple-dog households in the United States. The American Veterinary Medical Association estimates that one-third of the 35 million households included more than one dog. You may have a choice to get either a mature dog or a puppy. Sometimes you have no choice at all, such as if you and another dog owner decide to live together. But to have peace in your home, your dogs must get along with one another.

The Mature Dog

Acquiring a mature dog may be a better choice than getting a puppy.

- When you buy a mature dog, you can see exactly how it looks. You will know its adult size, and you will know if it has the physical characteristics that you admire.
- The mature dog you buy probably will already have had some training. It is likely that it is housebroken, and, if not, it is old enough to be housebroken in just a few days. Mature dogs are often over the worst of the chewing and destructive stages of their lives.

- Some adult dogs available for new homes will have had obedience lessons; a few of them even obey advanced commands. Most will walk on leash. Many are accustomed to being handled and groomed. You can check the level of training of a mature dog by running it through a few basic commands. If the dog *sits*, *downs*, and *heels* on command, much of its necessary training will have been done by its previous owner.
- The mature dog usually will have had veterinary care. Many are completely vaccinated and need only periodic boosters. Many are spayed or neutered. Many are negative for intestinal parasites and are on heartworm preventive medication. All this will save you time, trouble, and money. The uncertainty of puppyhood illnesses is eliminated when you buy a mature dog.
- If you want a working or a hunting dog, you can evaluate the potential of a mature dog much more accurately than you can judge the potential of a puppy. You never can be sure that a puppy will inherit its parent's desire to point, retrieve, or to herd livestock. If you want a show dog, you can tell by its conformation if the mature dog will be a winner.
- Acquiring a mature dog is a humane act. Mature dogs of almost every breed and all mixtures of breeds are literally dying for good homes. National rescue groups have many purebred dogs

that are available for a variety of reasons. City and county animal shelters are full of fine dogs needing homes, and many of these dogs will be put to death if they are not adopted. It is an act of compassion to buy one of these dogs and give it a chance to live.

You Can Make It Work!

It is not necessary for your dogs to love, or even like, one another for them to live in the same household. All that is required is for each of your dogs to tolerate the presence of the other without overt aggression. Even if they enter into an armed truce, if it is a durable truce, you will have peace.

In many ways, dogs are like children. The actions of children toward other children are governed by many

Four good friends.

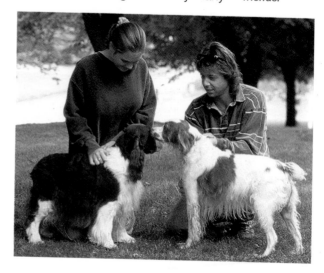

emotions: playfulness, jealousy, possessiveness, timidity, curiosity. Some children always play together happily, and share their toys, while some occasionally have little quarrels. Some cannot be together without fighting unless a parent is present. A few will pick a fight even in the presence of a parent. Children are quick to learn what they can get away with before a parent intervenes.

Many of our companion dogs are raised in an exclusively human society. They seldom, if ever, come into contact with other dogs. They do not know how to relate to members of their own species. It is unrealistic not to expect these dogs to exhibit hostility when a strange animal enters their territory.

Although dogs' behavior toward other dogs is governed both by instinct and by experience, they are quick to learn which of their actions will be tolerated by their owners. When you have more than one dog in your life, you must be the "parent" who establishes the rules of conduct for each of them.

Obedience Classes

Obedience classes are not merely a place where dogs learn to heel and stay; the classes are much more important in shaping dogs' behavior. In obedience classes, dogs learn that their owners' words require them to make specific responses. In good obedience classes with knowledgeable trainers, dogs learn that they have no choice but to respond to their owners' commands.

In obedience classes, dogs learn that they must respond to commands under the most distracting of circumstances: *in the presence of other dogs.*

When you plan to acquire another dog, take your resident dog or dogs to obedience school. By their reactions to the other dogs in the class, you will get a good indication of how they will behave toward your new dog. A dog that is eager to play with its classmates will more easily accept another dog in its family. A dog that is ready to fight in obedience classes will be even more ready to do battle with another dog in its home territory.

If your resident dog already has been to an obedience class, it may be a good idea to enroll it in a refresher course. If you get another dog before you have had time to take your first dog to a class, enroll it in one as soon as you can. You can teach it to obey your commands at the same time as you teach it to tolerate the new dog.

If possible, also enroll your new dog in an obedience class. If you have a family member or friend who can handle one dog, enroll both in the same class. This will give you a head start in training the two dogs to live together in peace.

Which Behavior Group Includes Your Dog?

In almost every case of aggression, your resident dog will be the one that is hostile toward other dogs that enter its territory. Your dog's degree of hostility will be that of one of the six behavior groups described in Chapter Four.

If your resident dog is in Group 1 (instant and total acceptance of other dogs), all you have to worry about is the possibility of overexuberant romping through your house. However, if your dog is in Group 6 (always shows murderous rage toward any other dog), be prepared to take strong measures to prevent fighting.

Once you have determined the behavior of your own dog, you have a starting point from which to achieve harmony in your multiple-dog household.

Controlling the Behavior of Your Resident Dog

Your resident mature dog will be in its own home territory so even if it is not aggressive toward other dogs, it is natural for it to express dominance over canine invaders. To prevent conflict that can escalate into serious fights, you must be in control of the actions of your own animal. As discussed (page 48), obedience school is a wonderful way to gain this control. You should also give your dog a short refresher course in the two lessons discussed in Chapter Three: the submissive position and the *down-stay*.

If your dog does not accept being placed in the submissive position without resistance, repeat the lesson until it does. This can mean anything from a single additional lesson to several lessons a day for as much as

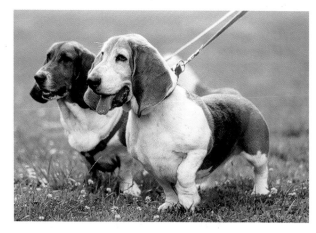

These two Basset Hounds have been friends for years.

a week. *If you cannot place your resident dog in the submissive position and hold it there without a struggle for as long as you like, you are not its leader. There is absolutely no way you will be able to prevent it from challenging another mature dog for a position of leadership.*

Unlike the submissive position, the dog must stay *down* without being held in place. Because this exercise is so restrictive, the *down-stay* is the cornerstone of control. You should be proud if you have a dog that will reliably *down-stay* in the face of extreme temptation. If your dog will not, it needs more training. It is up to you if you chose to accept the *sit-stay* instead of the *down-stay*. Remember, a dog feels much less restrained by the *sit* instead of the *down*, and will break position with much greater alacrity.

Learning about the New Dog

Even though the new dog will be at a disadvantage because it is entering a strange environment, some new dogs will challenge the resident dog for dominance. If you can discover some facts about your new dog, you will have a good idea what to expect.

- Was your new dog an only pet? It might not have learned to accept the presence of another animal, and might automatically be hostile toward any other dog. If it is, a fight will ensue unless your first dog is an absolutely accepting and submissive Group 1 animal. Even if your first dog will not fight back, it might be badly injured by a hostile newcomer.
- Has your new dog had any submission handling or obedience training? Does it have any idea of the meaning of the words *"No!"* or *"Down"*? If not, you have little or no voice control over how it will act.

Often (but not always) you can talk to the former owners of your new dog and get answers to these questions. If you cannot, it will be worth your time to test the behavior of the new dog for yourself.

1. Take the dog to a quiet place and handle it all over, including its feet. If it offers to bite when you touch it, its actions toward your resident dog will not be under your control.
2. If the dog does not resent your handling it, try to place it in the submissive position. If it shows no resistance, you soon can gain control of its actions.

When you have determined the level of control you have over both the new and the resident dog(s), you will be prepared to establish a nonviolent relationship between them.

The New Dog's Own Sanctuary

When you obtained your resident dog, you established a *safe place* in which to keep it when you were not supervising its actions. By the proper use of its safe place, you taught your dog to be housebroken and to not be destructive in the house in your absence. In the majority of cases, your resident dog will have outgrown the need for its safe place; it will be trustworthy to allow loose in the house even when nobody is home.

Your new dog is in a strange environment. Even though many adult dogs are trained to not mess or damage anything in the house, this training might not carry through perfectly from its former home to yours. Establish a safe place for your new dog before you bring it home. Do not use the resident dog's place for your new dog unless you never use that place for the first dog. Do not arrange the two safe places where the dogs can see each other; confined dogs often will bark and snarl at all other dogs in sight. At least initially, try to have the places in different rooms.

One of the many advantages in getting a mature dog is that you may not have to establish a cagelike safe place for it. Depending on its temperament and training, a new mature dog might be safely confined in a small room such as a bathroom, or even in a bedroom. But if you know little or nothing about your new dog's previous life, it is much more satisfactory if you confine it in a place in which it cannot destroy anything of value.

Using the Correct Equipment

Both dogs—the resident and the newcomer—must wear equipment that will enable you to restrain them. If a dog can pull its head out of its collar or jerk the leash out of its handler's hands, it will be out of control. Loose dogs can cause serious damage, both to other dogs and to people.

As detailed in Chapter Five, the equipment needed to control a dog depends on the size of the dog, the disposition of the dog, and the strength of the handler. If you are introducing two Chihuahua puppies, two thin leashes and two buckled collars are more than adequate. If the dogs are both adult male Rottweilers, you might need a muzzle or a halter and a thick leash for each of them. Be ready to do the job right. *Do not try to introduce two dogs without adequate equipment.* All parties can be seriously hurt.

General Rules for Introducing Two Dogs to Each Other

Believe it or not, most dogs fall into Group 1 or 2. Your dog might put up a tremendous fuss the minute it sees another dog, but it is most likely

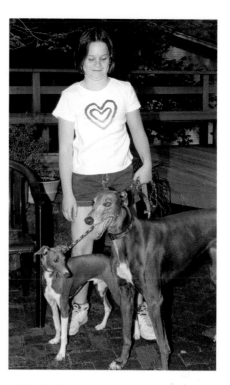

This owner keeps both of her dogs controlled on their leashes.

a bluff. Very soon, its curiosity will cause it to want to approach the new dog, to smell the new dog, and soon to romp with the new dog. However, even though you will have little trouble getting most dogs to accept one another, the process will be safer and easier if you follow the rules:

• Bring your new dog home and allow it to relax in its own safe place, out of sight of your resident dog. Exercise them separately the first few times. The dogs will be aware of the presence of one another by scent, and will not be taken by surprise when they meet. If you anticipate hostility, you might keep the dogs completely apart for a day or two.

Even scrappy Terrier breeds can live together.

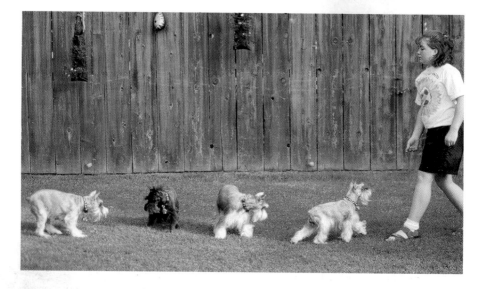

- Make the first introduction of the dogs outdoors. Your resident dog has an instinct to protect its home from intruders. All dogs have this instinct, no matter how friendly they seem. Even though your yard is part of your resident dog's territory, it is much larger than the relatively small area inside a room. Never make a dog feel trapped in a small space with a possibly hostile stranger.

   Little is accomplished by arranging the initial meeting of the dogs in an area that is strange to both dogs. When you take both dogs back to your own yard, your resident dog will display the same hostility, as if the dogs had never met.
- Keep both dogs on leashes until you are confident of their actions, even if your yard is fenced. Both dogs must be under control for the initial meetings. Try to have a helper hold the new one on leash while you control your resident dog's actions.
- Remove all objects from the environment that might cause competition. This means: Take away all balls, bones, toys, and food and water bowls, both in and out of doors. Always feed each dog in a separate location, and offer no treats until you are absolutely sure the dogs will not fight over them. In many multiple-dog households, each dog can have toys and treats only in its own safe place.
- Never try to placate a dog that is expressing hostility. Growling, barking, and snarling constitute misbehavior and should be corrected with at least a verbal reprimand. Soothing talk is interpreted by a dog as approval. Tell your growling dog *"No! No!"* Don't say, *"Good Boy"* or *"Good Girl."*

52

Introducing Dogs from Group 1, 2, or 3

- Handle the resident dog yourself for the introductions. Get a friend or family member to assist you by handling the new dog.
- Bring the new dog out of the house and have your assistant hold it on a leash. Then bring your resident dog outdoors and place it in a *down-stay* about 20 feet (6 m) from the new dog. Get a good grip on the leash. Ask your helper to approach to within 15 feet (4.6 m) with the new dog. Insist that your resident dog remains down, even if you have to hold it there. Remember, you are the leader and you will govern how the dogs will act. Have your helper lead the new dog back and forth while the resident dog watches it. Fortunately, in most cases the two dogs will express curiosity about each other, but will not express hostility. The dog most likely to be aggressive is the resident. If it shows hostility, continue to insist on the *down-stay* until the dog will pay more attention to you than to the strange dog. Insisting on the *down-stay* position inhibits a "bad" action (demonstrating aggression toward another dog) by substituting a "good" action (obeying the handler).

  If your resident dog does not seem hostile, allow it to stand and watch the other dog. If it shows no acts of aggression, allow the dogs to sniff one another but be sure that each handler keeps a tight hold on each dog's lead. Be ready to yank the dogs apart and place your first dog back in the *down-stay* position if it growls.
- Expect most dogs to be interested in each other. Dogs in Groups 1 and 2 will act playful. Those in Group 3 will simply act as if the other dog was not present. Dogs in Group 4 will growl or snarl at one another, but will respond to your command "*No! No!*"
- Allow both dogs, on leash, to walk around and observe each other. If neither is hostile, you are ready to take them into the house.
- Take the newcomer in first and let it walk around and smell the environment. Keep it on a leash, and have your assistant hold the leash.
- Bring the resident dog indoors on a leash. Control this leash yourself.
- In the relatively confined area indoors, each dog's hostility level will advance approximately one group. Dogs in Groups 1 and 2 are likely to react more cautiously to the interloper. Dogs in Group 3 that ignored each other outside probably will express more hostility when indoors. Keep both dogs on leashes and repeat the same procedure you used outside. Place the first dog in a *down-stay* while it watches the new dog. Then allow it to get up and approach the new dog. Allow them to sniff each other.
- After a ten-minute introductory period, place the new dog in its safe place to relax. Allow your resident dog to resume its usual activities.
- Repeat the introduction procedure after an hour or so. For at least two

days, leave leashes on both dogs whenever they are together. Hold the leash of your resident dog if it seems at all hostile. Keep the new dog on leash, held by another person, for as long as needed. If the dogs seem reasonably compatible, you do not need to hold the leashes; let the dogs drag them. Dragging leashes serve as mental and physical restraints to dogs, and if necessary, the leashes will allow you to pull the dogs apart if one should start a scrap.

- If the dogs become overexcited, limit the length of time the dogs are together. A "time out" in its safe place may allow each dog to become more calm. When you resume the introduction, limit it to a few minutes. As they act less excited, gradually increase the time the dogs are together.

  Do not expect a dog to regard a "time out" in its safe place as punishment for unacceptable behavior. The interlude is merely an opportunity for each dog to relax.

- When you are comfortable with having both dogs together with dragging leashes, take them both outside, still on leashes. If your yard is fenced, you can hold the leash of your resident dog since it is much more likely to be the aggressor, and let the new dog's leash drag. If your yard is not fenced, you need to have the new dog tied to something or held by another person so it cannot run off or approach the resident dog. The dogs probably will interact

more peacefully outdoors than they did in the house.

Take the leashes off, one dog at a time, *only* when you feel entirely comfortable that the dogs will not fight. Take the leash off the most submissive dog first. This probably will be the new one.

- Both dogs will accept each other gradually. Do not try to hurry the process, but repeat the introductory sessions as often as you feel necessary. Your dogs' actions will tell you when it is safe to allow them to be together without restraint. When both the resident dog and the newcomer are in Group 1 or 2, it will take only a few days to achieve complete harmony; it may take a week until dogs in Group 3 tolerate one another.

Working Alone

All new owners will not have the luxury of an assistant to handle the new dog while they handle the resident. It is best if another handler can be present at least for the dogs' initial meetings, but, if necessary, you can accomplish the introductions by yourself.

- If you have nobody to help by holding the new dog on leash, you must substitute some form of passive restraint. When you take your new dog out of the house, chain it securely in your yard before you bring out your resident dog on leash. Use a chain instead of a rope or leash that the dog could chew.

  The new dog will be in a strange place, which will inhibit any aggressive tendencies it may have. When your resident dog is brought out, some new dogs will stand and wag their tails. Some will ignore the resident dog. Some will lunge to the end of their chains and bark. Ignore them. Place your resident dog in a *down-stay* 15 or 20 feet (4.6–6 m) away. When the new dog stands quietly, you can allow your resident dog to approach to about 15 feet (4.6 m) before resuming the *down-stay*. If both dogs seem friendly, allow them to sniff each other.

- If you are handling the meeting alone, you will have to take your resident dog in the house and confine it before you bring in the new dog. Tie the new dog securely in a room, and proceed as though it were being held on leash by another person. Arrange for several meetings between the dogs before you release the new one, always tying your new dog before you bring in the resident dog on leash. This will enable you to yank your resident dog away if it acts hostile.

- An easy way to tie a dog in the house is to attach a short piece of rope onto the end of its chain and close the rope in a door that latches securely. Tie a knot in the rope on the outside of the door so that the dog cannot pull the rope out of the jamb. You can use a leather or cloth leash instead of a chain if your new dog is not likely to chew it.

- When you are ready to allow your dogs more freedom together, release the leash on the least aggressive one while you restrain

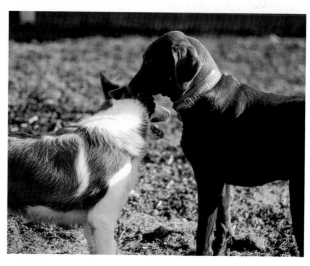

the other. Then allow both dogs to drag their leashes, and finally to interact without restraint.

The Border Collie makes friends with the Labrador Retriever.

Introducing a New Dog from Group 4 or 5

Dogs that are in Group 4 or 5 are those that express mild to strong aggression toward a strange dog. They growl and snarl; hair stands up on their backs; some resist being forced to assume the *down-stay* position.

Many dogs act as though they are in Group 4 or 5, when they are actually in Group 2 or 3. They will start out barking and leaping around at the sight of another dog, but soon will be willing to wag their tails, sniff each other, and initiate play behavior.

Use the same procedure to acquaint dogs in Groups 4 and 5 as you would if the dogs were in Group 1, 2, or 3, but you must repeat the introductory meetings on leash many more times. This may take days, or even weeks. Only when neither dog growls or threatens the other should they be allowed to sniff; only when they sniff each other peacefully should they be allowed to drag their leashes; only when you are sure they will not fight should the leashes be removed.

Arranging Introductory Meetings

Many short introductory meetings are far better than a few long ones. Each new time two dogs see each other is a new occasion to learn to interact without hostility. Eventually, most dogs' hostile behavior will disappear. Remember, every dog is an individual. Only time will determine how many controlled meetings are necessary before the dogs tolerate each other.

When the New Dog Is the Only Aggressor

The new dog is at a disadvantage since it is entering an environment that the resident dog considers to be its own, but if the first dog is of a submissive temperament and the new dog is in Group 4 or 5, the newcomer may be the troublemaker.

The new dog will not be under your control, since the two of you have not been together very long. What can you do?

1. Immediately institute a training program for the new dog. Obedience lessons, formal obedience school, and submission training will bring the dog under your control.

2. Hold the new dog on leash and have the resident dog restrained by another person or on a secure chain to prevent its approach. Allow closer contact only when the new dog ceases to demonstrate aggression.

3. Keep the new dog restrained whenever the resident dog is present. If the resident dog is cautious of the other, you can allow it to be loose during these sessions. You might have to keep the aggressive dog on a leash for weeks until it demonstrates that it will obey you and maintain the *down-stay* position in the presence of the resident dog. When the new dog is under your control, let it get up and drag its leash while in the presence of the first dog. That way, you can pull it away if it acts in an aggressive way.

Chapter Eight

The Tough Customers: Dogs in Group 6

Chapter Four explained which dogs are most likely to be in Group 6, those dogs that exhibit murderous rage at the sight of any other dog. Many dogs that seem to demonstrate this behavior are not genetically in Group 6, but are dogs that have seldom or never had contact with other dogs—they really do not know how to relate to another of their species. Once the shock of the initial contact is over, these dogs usually show the behavior of dogs in Group 4 or 5, occasionally even that of dogs in Group 2 or 3. If your dog acts like a Group 6, assume that it will attack until proven otherwise.

Take no chances; dogs with Group 6 behavior will seriously maim or kill other dogs, and will bite humans who attempt to prevent or separate their attacks. If you have a Group 6 dog, decide how you will handle the situation *before* you bring another dog home.

- A Group 6 dog may never be trustworthy with another dog in the absence of its owner. A few dogs in this group will never be trustworthy even when the owner is present. Be prepared to exercise caution every time such a dog is in the presence of another animal.
- Group 6 dogs usually respond poorly to discipline by their owners. Consider an intense course of obedience training for your Group 6 dog before you acquire another dog. *Intense* involves professional help—such as an obedience class taught by an experienced trainer—and twice-daily practice sessions.

These two dogs are unwilling to share the same turf.

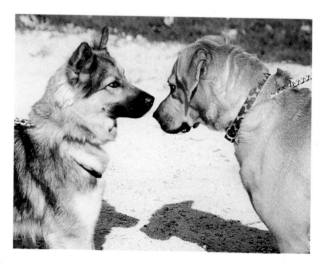

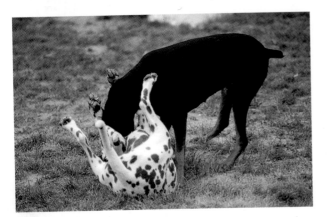

Never allow two dogs loose together until you are sure they won't fight.

Controlling Aggression

The key to controlling the aggression of a Group 6 dog toward another dog depends on these two factors:

1. the owner's ability to enforce the command "*Down, stay*," and
2. the owner's eternal vigilance whenever the Group 6 dog is not physically restrained in the company of other dogs.

If your resident dog is a Group 6, don't even try to introduce the new dog for a few days. Exercise each dog separately in the yard and allow each dog separate time loose in selected rooms of the house. That way, each dog will become familiar with the scent of the other before they meet.

If you feel confident that you can physically control your resident Group 6 dog and your helper can physically control the new dog, you can bring them out into the yard together. Do not allow them to approach each other closer than about 20 feet (6 m). Large, strong dogs can lunge at one another surprisingly quickly. *Do not take chances*—keep them well apart.

Intense does not include any form of mistreatment of the Group 6 animal.

- Ninety percent of Group 6 dogs are males; you may be more successful if your new dog is a female. Group 6 dogs are almost all over two years of age; consider acquiring a puppy. A castrated Group 6 dog may be a little more amenable to discipline and more likely to accept another dog than one that is intact; however, castration is not a cure-all; it will not completely change a dog's genetic or learned behavior.
- Remember: Group 6 dogs will attack and kill females and pups as well as males and older dogs, although they are more likely to eventually accept them.
- If your Group 6 dog gets loose and can reach another dog, it will attack. Prepare a separate secure enclosure for each of your dogs.
- Never try to introduce a Group 6 dog to another dog when you are alone unless you exercise special precautions. Always have a person or a stout barrier to restrain each dog.

Enforcing the *Down-Stay*

The handler of the new dog should hold it in a relatively small area, preferably without it barking or jumping around. You, the owner, should enforce your resident dog to assume a *down-stay*. This will not be easy, and some Group 6 dogs will redirect their aggression toward their

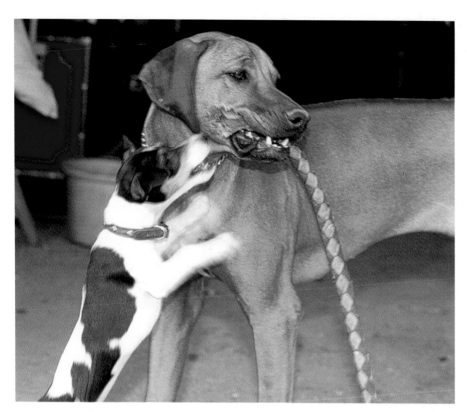

handlers. Control your dog with a head halter or a cone-type muzzle (see Chapter Five).

After five minutes of *down-stay*, take your resident dog out of sight. Wait a half-hour and let the dogs see each other, again outdoors. If you are successful in enforcing the *down-stay*, bring the dogs a few feet closer to each other and increase the time of the down-stay to up to ten minutes. Confirmed Group 6 dogs will need days or weeks of such introductions and very gradually diminishing distance between the animals before they will no longer attempt to attack the newcomer.

Even when the resident dog is willing to stay in the *down* position in the presence of the other dog, presume that it is biding its time until it can attack. Release it from the *down-stay* by giving it another command ("*Heel*") rather than your regular release command ("*Okay*"), which theoretically would allow it the freedom to approach the other dog.

The Resident Dog's Safe Place

The absolute worst way to introduce a Group 6 dog to another is to allow the new dog to approach when the resident is confined to its safe place. When in confinement, even a Group 2 or 3 dog will bark and snarl at the approach of another. Instead, lead your resident Group 6 dog to a place from which it can see the new-comer in its own safe place. Command "*Down, stay,*" and enforce the command for five minutes. Command "*Heel,*" and lead your Group 6 dog out of the room. Repeat this encounter many times, over many days. Gradually decrease the distance and increase the time that your resident dog is required to stay down while observing the new dog in its safe place. When you finally bring the resident dog into the presence of the new dog out of its safe place, be sure that the new dog is held on leash or securely chained. Many dogs are astonishingly incautious about approaching another dog that will harm them.

Avoiding a Dogfight

You can never be too cautious. Fighting dogs can cause each other permanent damage, even death. Never assume that your Group 6 dog is reformed; always suspect that it is just waiting for its chance to attack. Exaggerating its aggressive tendencies is far safer than false confidence in its benevolent behavior.

When you have a Group 6 dog and acquire another dog, keep both of them on leash for days or weeks after neither dog has demonstrated aggression toward the other. When you remove the leashes, do it cau-

Don't Get Hurt!

People can be horribly mauled by dogs. Never take a chance that you will be bitten, on purpose or by accident. If a fight does occur, never try to separate the combatants with your body. Grab something, anything, to thrust between the fighters. In the house, a chair is useful for this purpose. Outside, use anything handy. When dogs are fighting with one another, the rule of never striking them is suspended; hit either or both of the fighters with anything you can find, while screaming "*DOWN! DOWN!*" at the top of your voice.

When you get them apart, be extremely cautious about grabbing either dog. They may not realize that they are no longer being attacked by the other dog, and may bite you.

tiously one dog at a time, starting with the least aggressive one.

Remember, new situations might stimulate aggression. Be cautious in the presence of a third dog and in a smaller space such as an automobile. Avoid the presence of food, toys, or any objects that may cause competition.

Note. Some dogs, usually large-breed males, will never become trustworthy around other dogs even in the presence of their owners. If you find that your dog is one of these, consider owning one dog only, or be resolved to keep them apart forever.

Chapter Nine

The New Puppy and Your Old Dogs

More than 75 percent of owners who acquire a new dog choose a puppy. Many owners select a breed, locate breeders, and choose a puppy from those offered for sale. Some people visit a shelter or a pet shop, or answer an advertisement in the newspaper. Owners may even buy a puppy on impulse. They may not actually select their puppy, but accept one that is in need of a home.

When a puppy enters a home in which there are other dogs, its owners face new problems. Not only do the owners have to train the puppy to be a successful house dog, but they must train it in a society that already includes one or more adult dogs. A few special training tips will make the job easy.

Training Tips

Establish the Puppy's Own Safe Place

If your resident dog uses a safe place, your new puppy must also have its own. If you have eliminated your older dog's safe place, you can use the old cage or enclosure for the puppy. Place it in a different location unless the older dog *never* sleeps or eats in the old location. An older dog that discovers a pup in its place may show severe territorial aggression.

If possible, locate your pup's safe place out of sight of the area in which you feed your older dog. Feed the pup only in its safe place. Dogs should never feel that they have to compete for their own food.

Protect Your Puppy

In every case, the dominant animal in a new puppy-resident dog relationship will be the older dog. This is the animal that has the advantage of status conferred by age and familiarity. Even though your resident dog may seem to be very accepting of the puppy, there are circumstances in which it might harm the pup:

• *If the resident dog is actively hostile to the pup.* Even though a puppy is seldom considered by an adult dog to be a challenge to its

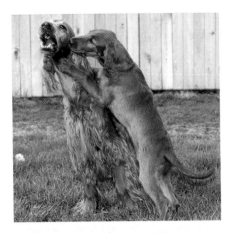

status, many dogs will resent a puppy that enters its territory. Some resident dogs will attack puppies and adult dogs alike.

- *When the puppy's attention is not wanted by the other dog.* If your new pup insists on jumping on the resident, it could get a bite from even the most mild mannered of older dogs.
- *When the older dog plays too rough.* The puppy may be too small and too submissive to withstand the playful actions of an adult dog.
- *When the puppy approaches the other dog's food dish, toys, or favorite sleeping place.* Dogs that seem to accept a puppy may be extremely competitive if the pup approaches their private property.

Leash-train Your Puppy as Soon as Possible

Most puppies are trusting little creatures. Your new pup will rush up to meet your resident dog, heedless of the possibility that the dog may

not be friendly. Until the puppy is trained to walk on a leash, you have no choice but to restrain it by holding it in your arms, or by kneeling and holding it in place on the ground.

Do not attempt to leash-train your puppy at the same time as you introduce it to your resident dog. If you hold the puppy on a leash before it has learned the meaning of the restraint, it will be frightened and struggle against the leash. For a puppy, each lesson should have only one objective: either to become acquainted with another dog, or to learn to respect restraint with a leash. Do not try to teach two lessons at the same time.

The puppy must learn that the leash will not harm it, and that when it is wearing a leash, its range is limited to the length of the leash. Most puppies learn this in one or two lessons.

When the pup is comfortable in your home, alternate ten-minute sessions of leash training with ten-minute sessions of dog-and-puppy introduction. For the first few days, you will need to restrain the puppy with your hands for the introductory sessions. You will be able to restrain your puppy more easily once it has learned to accept the leash.

Leash-training a puppy is simple.

Step 1. Fit the puppy with a lightweight buckled collar. The puppy will try to grab the collar with its mouth and to scratch it off with a hind foot. Be sure to fasten the collar tight enough so that the puppy cannot get its lower jaw under it. Leave the collar on the puppy at all times, so that the pup can become accustomed to it. Check that there are no projections in the puppy's safe place onto which the collar could be caught when you are not watching.

Step 2. Start to leash-train the puppy indoors where there are few distractions. Allow the puppy to wear the collar for a few hours to get used to it. Take the puppy out of its safe place and tie a 6-foot (1.8 m) piece of light rope to its collar. Use your good leash only if you do not mind if the puppy chews on it. Let the puppy play, dragging the rope, until you are sure that the puppy is not frightened by the rope. Most puppies will consider it a new toy.

Step 3. Get a handful of tiny, delicious treats for the puppy, something special that the puppy does not receive at its regular meals. As previously mentioned, small cat treats are good for this purpose. Take one of these treats in your closed fist, kneel or bend down, and let the puppy smell it. Say: "*Fido, come*," open your hand, and let the puppy eat the treat. Back away, get another tiny treat, and repeat the action.

Step 4. When the puppy demonstrates that it is looking for the treat, stand up while you say: "*Come,*" and offer the treat. Do this several times so that the puppy learns that the command "*Come*" means that you will give it a bit of food when it gets to you. If you want your puppy to look at your face in anticipation of a verbal command, hold your fist and the treat up to your chin. Lower your hand only to present the treat. During

all this training, the puppy should be dragging the rope behind it.

Step 5. Pick up the end of the rope. *Coax,* never drag, the puppy to come to you for the treat, using small tugs on the rope, never hard yanks. If the puppy does not rush right over to you, bend down and show it the treat. Next, walk backward while coaxing the puppy to follow with your voice and the treat. Give the treat only after you and the puppy have taken several steps together.

Step 6. Turn and walk forward while coaxing. Offer the treat only after the puppy follows for quite a few steps. Walk from room to room, or around the dining room table, coaxing the puppy with your voice, small tugs on the leash, and an occasional treat.

Now and then, stop walking, stand still, and let the puppy roam to the end of the rope. Coax it back to you with tugs on the rope. Reward it with praise and a treat when it obeys. Soon the puppy will accept the restraint of the rope without resentment or fear, and will follow you willingly wherever you lead.

Step 7. Leash-train your puppy in other locations. When it shows that it understands leash restraint, take it on a leash to unfamiliar locations both indoors and out so it will learn to accept the leash under all conditions. If the puppy mouths or chews on the leash while you are walking, distract it with your voice or by changing your direction or speed. Do not punish the puppy for mouthing the leash. At this stage of

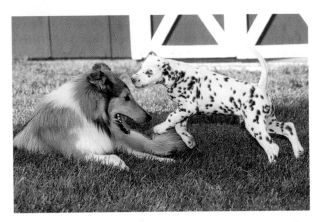

the education of the puppy, the leash is not to be associated with punishment of any kind. *Never lose your temper.* Do not advance to the next step until your puppy responds promptly to the previous one, even if it takes several training sessions.

If the puppy balks or pulls back, never yank it to you. Stop, turn to face it, and *coax.* Kneel down if you must. Early leash training should be accomplished with praise and reward, never with discomfort and fear. You are establishing a foundation for all the behaviors you will teach your puppy throughout its lifetime. Make it fun!

A puppy can concentrate on only one thing at a time. Hold your puppy on leash when you introduce it to your resident dog *only* when you are sure the pup is not frightened by leash restraint.

Make Introductions Carefully

Introduce your new puppy to your resident dog in a series of ten-minute sessions. At the conclusion of each session, return the puppy to

its safe place. If possible, arrange for three or four sessions a day. Allow at least an hour between each session.

Almost all pups, unless they are terribly fearful, will be members of Group 1. These pups will eagerly approach all other dogs, often to their detriment. Most adult dogs will act one group less aggressive toward a puppy than they will act toward another adult dog; in other words, dogs in Group 2 will behave toward a puppy as though they were in Group 1; dogs in Group 4 will act like members of Group 3. It is only resident dogs in Groups 5 and 6 that are a real danger to your pup.

Resident Dogs in Group 1 or 2

Get someone else to restrain the puppy while you hold your resident dog on a leash. If you are not sure about how the older dog will act, it is best to have it wearing a head halter so you can control its jaws.

If the puppy is not leash-trained, have a helper kneel and hold it in one place on the ground. If the pup is leash-trained, have it wear a plain buckled collar with a leash, and ask your helper to keep it in a small area at his or her feet.

If your older dog is in Group 1 or 2, you may allow it to sniff the puppy, then allow your resident dog enough leashed freedom to interact with the pup, but keep control.

If your dog shows no aggression toward the pup, you can allow the puppy the freedom to approach it and even to institute play behavior.

64

Remember, it is the rare pup that will act in an aggressive way. Most puppies will approach the resident dog, jump on it, and lick its face. Keep your resident dog on its leash until you are sure of its behavior. Plan for a minimum of three ten-minute introductory sessions before you take the leash off the Group 1 resident, four or more sessions if the resident is in Group 2. If your dog accepts the pup, you may drop the leash, but be alert to grab it at the first sign of discord.

Resident Dogs in Group 3 or 4

It is highly unlikely that any adult dog in Group 3 will actually attack a puppy. Your Group 3 resident will probably sniff the pup, then go lie down in its own bed or corner. The resident will snap only if you permit the puppy to approach it or jump on it. If your puppy is leash-trained, restrain it from annoying the resident. If it is not, hold it to keep it out of harm's way. After the ten-minute session, return the puppy to its safe place. After a few such sessions, the puppy and dog will be accustomed to seeing each other—the puppy will be less excited by the presence of another dog and less inclined to bother it.

The Group 4 dog will not be willing to accept the puppy at first, but will be under control of your voice. You can tell it *"Down"* while you or your helper prevent the puppy from approaching. Keep the resident on leash for six or eight sessions, until

you are sure it has no intention of molesting the pup.

Resident Dogs in Group 5 or 6

Dogs in Group 5 or 6 are the ones that will harm your puppy. Group 6 dogs attack without even a pause to see if the new animal is an adult or a pup, dominant or submissive. You must keep dogs in these groups on leash, preferably with a head halter, whenever the two animals are in the same area. After weeks of introductory sessions, you may be able to drop the leash of the Group 5 animal. After a few more weeks, you may feel secure enough to remove its leash entirely.

It is entirely possible that it *never* will be safe to leave your Group 6 dog alone with your puppy, even when it has reached adulthood. The more mature your puppy becomes, the more likely your Group 6 dog is to attack it and the more likely the puppy is to fight back. Even toy breed members of Group 6 can do significant damage and can provoke another dog into retaliating in self-defense.

Protecting Smaller, Older, or Very Submissive Resident Dogs

If you allow it, your resident adult dog may have its life made miserable by your new puppy. A big

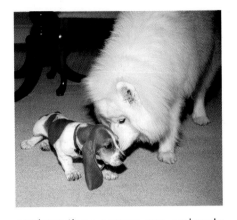

rambunctious puppy can seriously harm a little, old dog. If you have a small, old, or very submissive resident, do not allow the puppy to nip it, jump all over it, or take its toys. Keep the dog and puppy apart until you have established control over the puppy's behavior. You may have to keep them apart indefinitely except the times when you are present to supervise their actions. Your little, old dog is not going to get bigger or younger, but your puppy will grow and become more dominant.

Objects of Competition

Pick up all toys, bones, rawhides, food, and food dishes. Establish an additional location for a water bowl if the older dog shows any signs of guarding its water from the pup. The dog and pup may have bones and toys only when the other is not present. Even when the puppy is older, it is wise to restrict the availability of any object over which the dogs may fight.

If Your Puppy Is Fearful

A few puppies will exhibit extreme fear of your resident dog. Those that are afraid probably have had little contact with humans or other dogs, and are afraid of everything.
• Treat these pups gently.
• Keep your resident dog under control on a leash, away from the puppy.
• Allow the pup to approach the older dog when it feels confident. You will make the fearful puppy more bold toward other dogs by allowing it to become more bold toward humans.
• Handle it often and offer treats from your hand.
• Never force it into a terrifying situation.

Chapter Ten
Conflict Among Resident Dogs

Attitudes of both dogs and humans change with time. Your two dogs might seem to be the best of friends for months, but one day, young Fido approaches Rover's rawhide chew toy. Without warning, Rover turns on Fido and bites him viciously.

Or, young Fido never disturbed Rover's dinner. All of a sudden, Fido gobbles his own food, then reaches for Rover's. Rover slinks away. What happened to cause these changes in the dogs' behavior? How are owners to know if their dogs will fight?

Change in the dogs' attitude toward each other seems to owners to occur without warning, but signs of impending conflict usually occur for months without owners noticing. Had they realized what was happening to their dogs, the owners could have taken appropriate precautions to avoid fights. When owners are aware of the factors that act to determine a dog's social position, they can be ready to take appropriate steps to prevent conflict that may escalate into outright aggression.

Changes in Social Status

Owners who have households that include two or more dogs, even if all the dogs are of similar ages and sizes, should be alert for changes in their dogs' behavior toward each other.

Two dogs and one Frisbee — a recipe for disaster.

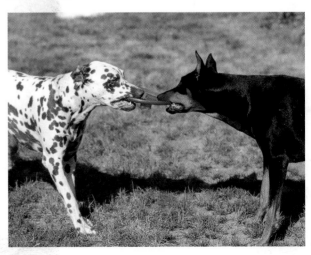

- One dog, usually the older, is the leader in each household. If the leader is not a dominant animal, this may not always be apparent. If the dog that has been the leader starts to be shoved out of the most favorable positions—first out the door, closest to the owner's chair—the dogs' status is changing.
- Dogs in a stable relationship do not growl at one another. Each member of the society accepts its position, so there is no need to growl a challenge. Dogs that are in a changing relationship growl warnings of their intentions to dominate or their refusal to submit. The owner who starts to hear growls soon will be hearing snarls, then seeing fights.

   Note. Play-growling is the exception to this rule. Dogs can growl in play without intending to dominate.
- Owners should recognize more subtle signs that one dog is challenging the other. The challenger may approach the other with a stiff-legged stare. The challenger's tail may be held stiff and may swish back and forth (not wag) at the tip. The hair over the challenger's back may stand on end. When owners recognize these signs, they can intervene before the challenge escalates into snarling and biting.

Reasons for Changes in Status
- The most common change is caused by the advent of social maturity. Puppies reach this stage at 18 months to two years of age. Social maturity has nothing to do with sexual maturity, which is reached at six to nine months old. Males and females, neutered or spayed, reach social maturity at about the same time in life.

   Until it reaches social maturity, the puppy or the adolescent dog will accept its submissive position to older dogs. When it becomes mature, the dog may no longer be willing to do so and may challenge the older dog for social supremacy.

   In the examples given, Fido, the younger dog, was submissive to Rover until Fido was two years old. Until that time, old Rover did not feel that his position in the family was challenged.

   As Fido became mature, subtle differences appeared in his attitude toward Rover. No longer did Fido follow Rover out the door; sometimes he pushed ahead to be first. No longer did Fido get up and walk away when Rover approached a favorite sleeping area; Fido stayed where he was and Rover walked away. If Rover is willing to accept the submissive role, the relative social positions of the dogs will become reversed: Fido will take over as top dog and Rover will be relegated to second place. If Rover strives to maintain his status and Fido does not back down, the dogs will fight. Two animals that once lived in harmony may become bitter enemies.
- Old age also affects the way in which dogs act toward each other.

As a dog becomes less vigorous, a stronger dog may successfully take over the older one's social position.

- Size and strength may play an important part. Dogs of the same age, even from the same litter, may be different in size. The larger will often dominate the smaller.
- Some breeds of dogs are genetically more likely to be dominant than others. For example, guard dog breeds will often dominate hound breeds.

Learned Behavior

When a large puppy pounces on a very small older dog, one of two things may occur. The puppy may receive a good nip and learn to respect the smaller dog, or the small dog may be frightened and run away. If the puppy is bitten, it may again challenge the older dog when the puppy reaches social maturity. If the small dog runs, there will be no challenge. The puppy has learned from the start that it can dominate the smaller, older dog, and the older dog has learned that it is not the boss.

There are circumstances in which a dog may be motivated to express aggression beyond its normal behavior. A mother dog with puppies, or a dog with a delicious bone, may protect the pups or property with such determination that other dogs will back away. Even though initially fearful, the protective dog may learn to accelerate its aggression to the point where most other dogs will avoid a challenge.

How Owners Can Keep the Peace

- *Be alert for signs of conflict.* Watch for changes in dogs' behavior toward each other. Recognize the warning signs before a fight breaks out and one or both dogs are injured.
- *Remove sources of conflict whenever possible.* Feed each dog in its own place. If they are fed in the same room, stay in the room to prevent the dominant dog from approaching the other's food. Pick up the dishes when the dogs are finished eating. Dogs seldom have conflict over water bowls, but have more than one source of water if necessary.
- *Do not allow food-type toys* (real bones, rawhides, chews) where more than one dog is present. Give these treats, if at all, only in each dog's safe place. Remove even non-food type toys such as

The puppy will not really challenge the older dog.

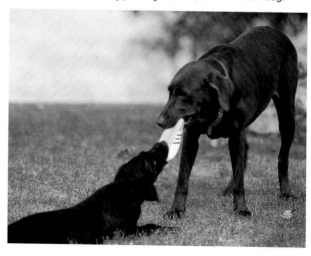

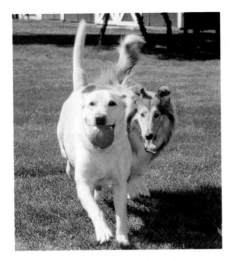

Will the Collie fight for possession of the ball?

rubber balls when the dogs are unsupervised.

- *Have your dogs under voice control.* If your dogs will not instantly obey the stern command, *"Down,"* practice until they will. At first, practice with each dog individually, then with both dogs together. Dogs that are under voice control can be prevented from attacking before they do serious damage. Dogs that are not under voice control can inflict many damaging bites before their owner is able to separate them.
- *Do not leave two dogs together in a confined space; do not leave two dogs together in a small space that contains food or toys.* Owners have had dogs that seemed to love to be together in a single safe place or in a small room. Suddenly, they find that one or both dogs have serious bite wounds on their bodies. Dogs need enough room to escape from one another if either becomes aggressive.

- *Be careful when you take more than one dog in a car.* The excitement of the ride may trigger aggression that would not occur at home. A minor dogfight in a moving vehicle can cause a serious accident. The environment in a car is exciting to dogs; excited dogs are more likely to start a scrap. Even if you take another person along, dogs that are able to reach one another may fight.
- If you are at all unsure of their conduct, separate your dogs when you leave them. Lock each in a different room or in its own safe place. Never allow the health—and certainly not the life—of one of your dogs to depend on the good nature of the other.

Dogs in Automobiles

If you must transport more than one dog at a time, try to enclose at least one of them in a carrier, crate, or cage. If you cannot enclose one of them, it is safer to transport two dogs in a station wagon or four-door sedan. Close the leash of one dog in the back door on the left side, and close the leash of the other dog in the front door on the right side. Be sure that the leashes are short. Tie a knot in each leash on the outside of the car so that a strong dog cannot pull its leash into the car.

If you are not sure the dogs are safely separated, make two trips. Avoid an accident at all costs.

Chapter Eleven

Cats: Prey or Pack Members?

Sixty percent of all dog-owning households in the United States are also home to one or more cats. In the majority of instances, both species exist with each other and with their human family members in relative harmony. In a few cases, open warfare prevails.

Cats are not small dogs. The hereditary social behavior of the feline species, *Felis domestica,* in no way parallels human or canine social behavior. Humans and dogs are, by nature, social animals. They live in communities of others of their species. Leaders and followers exist within these communities. The distinction between leaders and followers is not absolute; leadership may fluctuate within the community depending on the circumstances. In both human and canine societies, leadership may be shared by more than one individual and may be yielded to an individual that proves itself to be stronger or more determined than its fellows.

The natural organization of both wild and domestic feline society is not at all the same as the organization of canine and human society.

Solitary Lifestyle of Cats

Domestic cats and almost all wild felines live solitary lives. Wild felines live and hunt alone. They associate with one another only at breeding time and before their family groups are old enough to disperse. The most notable exceptions to this rule are African lions, which live in small groups called prides. African lions hunt in packs for the large ungulates upon which they feed. Undoubtedly, it is the large size of lions' prey species that led them to enter into group behavior. Most other feline species prey upon animals small enough to be captured by a single animal.

The solitary nature of the domestic cat may be disputed by the argument that groups of cats within a household often are on friendly terms with each other. This behavior actually resembles that of a family of

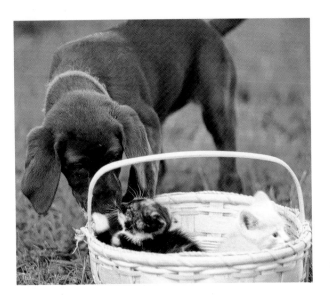

Young animals, even of different species, are not likely to attack each other.

own "pack," or must be taught that preying upon cats is forbidden. Cats must learn that the dogs in their own household are harmless to them.

Adding a Cat to Your Household of Dogs

You have had dogs for years. You always wanted a cat, and the neighbor's kittens are big enough for new homes. Is now the time?

Introducing a Kitten and a Puppy

A puppy that has had no experience with cats will consider your new kitten to be another playmate. Your job will be to prevent the puppy from harming the cat unintentionally, as well as to prevent the cat from scratching the pup's eyes out, quite intentionally. Restrain your puppy on a leash in a closed room, while you allow the kitten to walk around. You need not reprimand the puppy for its curiosity; just prevent it from rushing up to the cat. If you get an adult cat or a big kitten, allow the pup to approach it where the cat can get away, such as by jumping up on a chair. Each animal will examine the other, and eventually accept or decide to ignore one another. If your puppy is too young to respond infallibly to the *down* command, keep it on a leash until you are sure it will not try to play too roughly with the cat. Instead of "teaching the pup a

immature wild felines before they become old enough to establish individual territories. Large congregations of feral cats can be found in the wild only where people put out food for them, just as large congregations of wild bears (also solitary animals) are found only at dump sites where they forage for food.

Relationship of Predator to Prey

The reason for dog-cat incompatibility is the relationship of predator to prey. Dogs are instinctively programmed to pursue animals smaller than themselves; cats instinctively run from animals that might kill them. To own both species without danger to either, these attitudes must be changed. Dogs must learn to accept cats as members of their lesson," an adult cat or a big kitten can do permanent harm if it scratches a curious pup's eyes.

Do not take the leash off your puppy unless the kitten is big enough to escape the pup's unwanted attentions. A rambunctious puppy can kill a small kitten without meaning it any harm.

Introducing a Cat to an Adult Dog

When you add a kitten or a cat to your household containing an adult dog or several adult dogs, you must be more careful to keep each of the animals safe from the others. Unless your dog is a young puppy, it will not regard your new feline as merely another dog. It will consider any cat you obtain as an animal of prey, an intruder in its territory, or an object of curiosity. Before you bring the cat home, try to picture how your dog will react.

The Size of Your Dog

One bite from a Rottweiler can kill a kitten, while many shrill barks and nips from a Chihuahua may not even discourage a bold cat. Consider the size as well as the dispositions of both parties when you plan your dog-cat introduction. Chapter Five will help you select the correct restraint equipment for your dog.

The Scent of Each Animal

When you introduce a cat into your household that contains dogs, it is a good idea to assign a room to the cat or kitten. Keep its bed, litter-box, and food and water dishes in

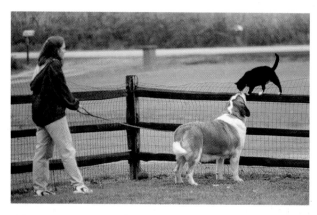

this room, and exclude the dog or dogs from the room for a day or two until the cat starts to feel at home. Your dogs will detect the scent of the cat, even several rooms away.

Once the cat has had a chance to feel comfortable in its new home, take it into another room from which the dogs are temporarily excluded. Allow the cat to explore the new area for a short time, then return the cat to its own room and admit the dogs to the room in which the cat has been. If you think that your dogs will be seriously hostile to the cat, repeat this scent introduction daily for two or three days. Each animal will become familiar with the presence of the other by its scent before the two actually meet.

Indoor Introductions

Dogs are less likely to chase, and cats are less likely to run within the boundaries of a closed room, if only because the area is smaller. Make your initial introductions in the room in which the animals have become familiar with the other's scent (see

If you are not sure of your dog's behavior, keep it on a leash.

Determine the Nature of Your Resident Dog

1. Do you have a puppy or a young dog that has had no experience with cats? You will have an easy job acquainting it with your new kitten or cat. All you have to do is to see that they do not injure one another.

2. Is your dog a hunter? Does it want to chase and catch other animals? Predatory behavior is common in most of the hunting breeds, as well as among the terriers. Dogs that are eager to chase balls and sticks are often eager to chase anything that moves, which probably will include your new cat.

3. Is your dog very territorial? Is it combative toward the neighbors' pets when they wander into your yard? Does it bark fiercely at the meter reader? Guard dog breeds as well as others with strong protective instincts will regard your cat as an intruder to be attacked or driven away.

4. Does your dog want to play with other animals? Does it consider the dogs in its obedience class to be exciting new friends? Dogs with this attitude might harm your cat, but only by playing too roughly with it.

5. Do you have a dog with a don't-bother-me attitude toward other animals? Such dogs will not voluntarily approach the cat. If a cat goes near it, a dog with this attitude will sniff the cat, growl at it, and get up and move away from it. Only if your kitten decides to initiate play action will this dog present a danger to the cat at all.

6. Is your dog one of the few that is afraid of cats? Puppies that have been scratched or bitten by aggressive cats often learn to respect all felines. If your dog seems to fear your kitten at first, be careful—fearful dogs that feel cornered will usually fight back. If the kitten gets too close, the dog might do the kitten serious harm.

above). Keep the doors closed, and have at least one person present other than yourself.

Keeping Both Animals under Control

Have the dog on a leash. If your dog is large, it is an excellent idea to restrain it with a dog halter rather than a plain or a choke collar. It is much easier to prevent a dog from launching an attack when you can use the halter to close its mouth and turn its head away from its intended victim.

Close your new cat in a carrier. Under no circumstances should you hold an adult cat in your arms in a potentially frightening situation. You could be bitten and scratched as the terrified cat struggles to get away. Even if you hold a cat or a kitten wrapped in a towel, you may be bitten and scratched. You may even be forced to release the cat if it struggles violently. A loose cat tearing around the room while an aggressive dog lunges at it is a recipe for disaster.

If you have no cat carrier, you can use a makeshift arrangement, but it must be secure and it must allow the dog to smell and see the cat moving inside the container. A strong box with holes cut in it or a plastic laundry basket with a securely tied lid can substitute for a carrier for an adult cat. A plastic crate for milk cartons will be big enough for a small kitten.

How to Begin Introductions

1. Take your dog on a leash into the room. Sit down in a comfortable chair with the dog lying down beside you. Have someone else carry in the cat in the carrier and set it down at least 6 feet (1.8 m) away. The dog will try to get up and investigate the carrier. Enforce the *down-stay* for a few minutes. If neither the dog nor the cat seems to be too upset with the other (no growling, barking, or hissing), have your helper bring the carrier a little closer. Allow the dog and cat to smell one another while the dog is still in the *down* position. Do not allow the dog to break the *down-stay*—the dog must learn that it is under your control in the presence of the cat.

2. If the dog acts at all hostile, move the carrier containing the cat back a few feet and keep the dog in its *down-stay* position an extra minute or two. Then have your helper take the cat in the carrier back to its own room before you allow your dog off leash. If you repeat this procedure a few times a day, you will make swift progress. Eventually, the dog will learn to relax in the *down-stay* position even when the cat in the carrier is no more than 3 feet (91 cm) away.

3. If you have no assistant, place the cat (in the carrier) in the room before you enter with the dog. It will be a little more difficult to establish the *down-stay* with your dog when it sees the carrier, but it will serve the same purpose. If you have more than one dog to introduce to the cat, bring only one of them into the room at a time. When each of the dogs obeys you while in the presence of the cat in the carrier, you can try both of them together. If you think the dogs will be aggressive, ask another person to handle one of them on a leash.

4. When your dog will relax next to your chair in the presence of the carrier containing the cat, open the carrier door. Allow the cat to look out, and to walk out if it will. Correct your dog the minute it moves toward the cat. If you have no trouble keeping your dog in the *down* position, allow the cat to walk around and explore the room. Do not let it get within reach of the dog unless you are sure the dog is not going to grab it.

Unless you have a very aggressive dog, you and your dog will reach this point in two or three days. If your dog is likely to attack the cat, take as many days as necessary to feel comfortable that your dog will remain in the *down-stay* before you open the carrier door.

When the dog shows no inclination to break the *down* position and leap up after the cat, allow the dog to sit, then stand, then *slowly* approach to within 3 feet of the cat. Do not let it get any closer; command, "*Down!*" You are teaching your dog that it is never to get closer to the cat than 3 feet unless the cat itself initiates the approach.

If the cat retreats, do not allow the dog to go after it. Return the dog to the *down-stay* position next to your chair. Wait until the cat feels comfortable enough to walk around the room before you again allow the dog to stand and move toward it.

5. Next you will drop the dog's leash in the presence of the cat. Before you let go of the leash, arm yourself with a water pistol, a loud noise-maker, or a soda can full of pebbles or coins. In other words, have something with which you can startle the dog if it makes an aggressive move toward the cat. A water pistol is best—you can squirt only the dog. Noisemakers will also frighten the cat. Allow the leash to drag and keep the water pistol in your hand when you first permit the dog to stand and walk around in the presence of the loose cat. Correct the dog with the leash and the startle device the minute it starts to approach the cat.

After a few half-hour sessions, your dog should be willing to obey your instructions and stay away from the cat. If you feel sure of the dog's good intentions, you can remove the leash. But do not trust it completely!

Separate When You Cannot Supervise

Never trust your dog and cat together in a place where one cannot escape the unwanted attentions of the other. If one of your animals is too small or too weak to escape from the other, or if the area in which they are enclosed is lacking in escape routes for the weaker pet, do not allow them to be together in your absence. You may return to find that your smaller pet, usually the cat, has been harmed by the stronger one.

Never, never close two dogs in a small room with a cat: Two dogs are more likely to gang up and attack than is one dog alone; however, two cats will seldom gang up on one dog. Except for a mother protecting her kittens, cats will not often enter into a fight to protect another cat. Remember: Canines hunt in packs; felines hunt alone.

Training for the Cat-chasing Dog

Do you own a confirmed cat-killer? The dog that "hates" cats usually does so because it has an extremely strong predatory instinct that has not been modified by training. The cat-killer has had the exciting experience of chasing and killing small animals, which has reinforced its instinctive response to attack cats as a prey species. Be careful with such a dog—it might consider small dogs and children to be prey species as well as cats.

You can own cats even if you have a dog with a reputation for attacking cats. It will take time and effort, but you can train your dog not to bother cats *while you are present.* If you are not willing to separate the dog and cats when you are not present, you should consider owning either the dog or the cats, but not both. If you ever think you can trust such a dog, you will to be disappointed and your cats will be in danger.

The routine used to train a confirmed cat chaser is the same as that used to train any other dog, with these exceptions:

- Be sure that you can physically control your dog. Use equipment, usually a headcollar or halter, that will enable you stop the dog whenever it makes a wrong move toward a cat. Dogs that attack cats are usually of large breeds. If the dog can drag you by the leash, you cannot control its actions.

- Practice the *down* with no cat in the room until the dog will stay without resistance for at least ten minutes. It does not have to stay in your absence; you can sit next to it and hold the leash. The dog need not stay for the entire ten minutes

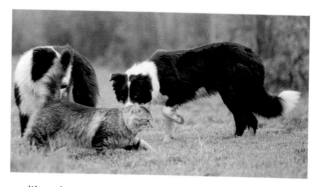

with only one command. If you see it start to move, repeat *"Down!"* as often as necessary.

- Be willing to take the time to enforce the *down* command dozens of times in the presence of the cat, first in the carrier, then loose in the room. If (or when) your dog tries to get up, correct it with the halter and place it back in the *down* position. It may take weeks of twice-daily lessons before your dog will not try to get up and grab the cat. Establish a warning command, such as *"No! No!"* or *"Ah! Ah!"* to discourage the dog before it makes a move. Don't give up— you can get it done!

Note. It is never appropriate to beat or otherwise mistreat your dog, even though it intends to do serious damage to your cat. Inflicting pain may cause your dog to intensify its efforts to attack the cat or to redirect its aggression toward you. You should correct the dog orally, even yell at it, as you replace it in the *down* position. You must be very firm, but never brutal. Make your corrections with the leash and headcollar, if possible. Shove

These Border Collies are herding the cat, not chasing it.

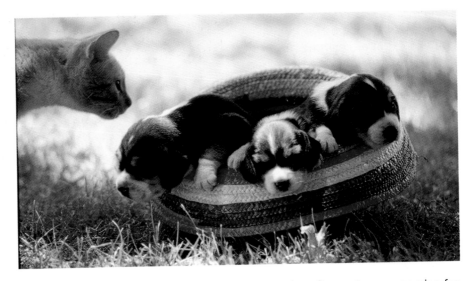

This cat is more curious than suspicious.

it down and hold it there, if necessary, until the dog will stay down even when the cat is loose.

- When you allow the dog to stand and walk around in the presence of the cat, keep the cat in the carrier the first few times. Only when the dog makes absolutely no move toward the carrier should you allow the cat to come out into the room. You will know your training is having the desired effect when the dog turns its head away and refuses to even *look* at the cat or the carrier. Beware of the dog that stares at the cat or tracks it with its eyes. A dog that watches the cat is considering attacking it. Do not trust this type of dog for many weeks off leash when a cat is present. Let the dog drag the leash until you feel sure you will not have to pull the dog away from the cat. Keep your water pistol handy.
- Never trust this dog with cats, indoors or out, in an unsupervised situation. Separate or supervise for the life of the dog and cat.

Adding a Dog to Your Household of Cats

Your cats will be afraid of your new dog or puppy. Cats' instincts insure that they do not approach unknown animals that can do them harm. Your cats will fear a strange new dog even though they may be good friends with your other dogs. Many cats will retreat to a safe place at the sight of a new dog, and not emerge until they feel more secure. It may be days until your cat crawls out from under the sofa when the new dog is present.

If your cat goes into hiding, place its food, water, and litterbox nearby. If the cat is afraid to come out to eat or drink, it will suffer. If it is afraid to approach its litterbox, it will eliminate somewhere else and your carpeting will suffer. It is best to establish a "dog area" and a separate "cat area" in your house. Eventually, each animal will become accustomed to the presence of the others and the areas will merge. This may take a month or more, but it will happen.

When Cats Are Aggressive

Cats have the instinct to protect their homes, just as dogs do. There are a few adult cats, usually males, that will demonstrate territorial aggression toward a newcomer by hissing and growling a threat, and even by attacking with teeth and claws. Never take the leash off your new dog until you have seen how your cat will act. If your cat is one of the few that will attack, you and the dog may suffer serious wounds until you get them apart.

Most cats that attack dogs do so from fear alone. A normal cat will try to get away from an unknown dog, but will fight fiercely if it feels cornered. Avoid a fight; never let this happen. Keep the leash on the dog and escape routes open for the cat until they are familiar with each other.

The New Dog May Harm Your Cats

You may get a dog with an actively predatory nature. Such a dog will try to attack your cats, even though it is in a new environment and the cats are in their home territory. You will be at a decided disadvantage to rectify

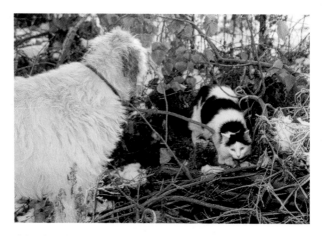

this situation because the dog is new to you and has not yet learned to obey your orders.

Never allow your dog to corner a cat.

If you know nothing about your new dog's behavior toward other animals, start its training days or weeks before you introduce it to your resident cats, keeping your pets apart until you have gained at least partial control over the new dog's actions. Practice until the average adult dog has learned to obey the *down* command with reasonable reliability. Then introduce it to the cats exactly as you would if the dog were the resident and the cats were the newcomers. If your new dog has a bad reputation around cats, take extra time to be sure that you can control the dog. Train your dog before it ever comes into contact with a cat, even a cat in a carrier. During this time, allow the dog and the cats alternate time in the same room. They will learn to accept the scent of each other, just as they did when you introduced a new cat to your resident dog.

Your Dog's Outdoor Behavior toward Cats

The dog that tolerates cats inside the house may chase, catch, and even kill those very same cats if both are loose outdoors. When dogs are not limited by the confines of a room or the close presence of humans, their predatory instinct may be stronger than their training. When this occurs, the dog will obey its instinct to chase and the cat will obey its instincts to flee. If it catches the cat, the dog may obey its instinct to kill. The dog that required strict measures to keep it from harming cats in the house should never be trusted off leash outdoors in the presence of cats.

The Litterbox

Since cats and dogs have such different social behavior, it is not surprising that they have different elimination behavior as well. House cats are expected to eliminate only in their litterboxes and dogs to eliminate only outdoors, but sometimes both species make mistakes. Often, dogs and cats eliminate where they should not because of the influence of other animals. Owners of both cats and dogs should plan ahead to avoid unpleasant problems.

Getting Safely to the Litterbox

No cat is so well trained that it will run past a dog that it fears to get to its litterbox. It will simply pick a spot it considers to be safe when it needs to eliminate, and the spot is unlikely to meet with a homeowner's approval. If your cat is afraid of your dog, it is absolutely essential that there be no obstacles to the cat getting safely to its litterbox. Remove even the obstacles that exist only in the mind of the cat. If there is a chance that a dog might inhibit a cat from getting to its box, relocate the dog. Do not let it lie in an area through which the cat must pass to reach its box.

If you are not able to assure that the dog will never be in the cat's path, relocate the litterbox or add more litterboxes. A cat that has learned to eliminate in a corner of the rug is hard to break of this habit.

Be sure that your cat feels safe once it has arrived at its litterbox. Even if it can get to the box easily, it will refuse to do so if it is afraid of a dog that might be in the area. If you have both cats and dogs loose in your house, the dogs often visit the vicinity of litterboxes because they are attracted by the odor.

Dogs and Cat Feces

Even though humans regard fecal material as disgusting, some other animals do not. It is the rare dog that will not eat cat feces, and it is the rare owner who is not entirely horrified to discover this. The reason that dogs eat cat feces is simple: they like the taste and smell.

The odor of the fecal material of every animal depends in part on the diet of the animal. To dogs, cat feces smell like cat food, which most dogs love. In fact, the accepted way to administer medication to a reluctant canine is in a piece of meat-flavored or fish-flavored cat food.

Eating cat feces might harm your dog if your cat has certain internal parasites that can be transmitted in its feces. Also, eating cat feces will give your dog severe, if temporary, halitosis.

Another problem arises when your dog waits for your cat to go to the litterbox to defecate so that it can grab the feces. If your cat fears that a dog will pounce on it, the cat will avoid the litterbox and defecate somewhere else.

It is not easy to keep your dogs out of the litterbox. You cannot make cat feces less attractive to your dogs by changing the cat's diet. Cats require the high-protein, high-fat content of cat foods to be healthy.

If your cat covers its stools with litter, you could try using a scented litter that *may* repel your dog. If you try this, be sure the scent does not also repel your cat. You could also use a covered cat box; however, some cats may be afraid to enter a covered box so leave the box uncovered until the cat is accustomed to using it, then put the cover over only part of the box at first.

If possible, find a location for your cats' litterbox that your dogs are unable to reach. A seldom-used bathtub is a good place; the cats can jump in and out, but few dogs are large enough to get into a litterbox inside a tub. You could put the litterbox in a basement or utility room and exclude the dogs by keeping the door partly closed with a brick. Do not count on training your dog with punishment not to get into the litterbox. It will learn not to do it when you are present, but will sneak into the box when your back is turned.

Scent-marking

It is a well-known fact that unaltered animals tend to mark their areas by urinating in many locations within the territory. It is less well known that some altered dogs and cats will also scent-mark as an expression of dominance toward other animals. Cats that express dominance by urine-marking may spray urine onto a vertical surface or simply deposit it on the floor.

When you find urine in the wrong places, one animal is telling you that it wants to elevate its social status in relation to the others. Presuming that all your animals are neutered and sex is not the stimulus for the marking, the best remedy is to confine the perpetrator to its own area unless it is under supervision. It is possible that the animal doing the marking will learn to accept its social position. Until then, separate or supervise!

Chapter Twelve

Birds, Rodents, and Other Caged Pets

Dogs are carnivores; they eat meat. Dogs' ancestors existed only by killing and eating other animals. It is irrational to expect dogs to ignore small creatures when their instinct tells them that these animals are *food.*

Domestication has weakened the predatory instincts of some dogs to the point that they will not even chase mice. Training has convinced a few dogs that their owners do not want them to pursue other animals.

Child, kitten, puppies, and dwarf rabbit all get along with each other.

Is your dog one of these? Do you have a dog with no hunting instinct? Have you trained your dog so well that it will not attack a prey animal? The lives of your small pets are at stake—don't bet on it!

There is only one safe way to keep dogs and small caged animals in the same household—*apart!* The dog that is only curious can upset a cage and destroy its inhabitants just as quickly as the dog that is actively seeking its natural prey. If you own both dogs and caged pets, you must take steps to prevent tragic accidents.

Taking Precautions to Prevent Tragedies

Place Cages in Safe Locations

Picture yourself in an elevator on the fourth floor. Imagine that the elevator cable breaks and the elevator plummets to the basement. What happens to you?

You and the elevator fall the equivalent height of four floors, the elevator is smashed, and you are maimed or killed. Even if you escape serious injury, you are bruised, shaken, and terrified. That is what happens to a small pet when a dog knocks down its cage. It can be worse if the cage breaks apart and the occupant escapes, only to be killed by the dog or lost in the house. Take the necessary steps.

- Place cages high out of dogs' reach. Owners of large dogs should avoid locating cages at tabletop height. Hang cages from the ceiling or place them on upper shelves.
- Avoid flimsy cage stands that are easily upset, even by small dogs. Discard the unstable stand that came with your cage and place the cage on a stronger base.
- Prohibit dogs' access to rooms containing cages. Owners of pets such as rabbits and ferrets often use cages that are located on the floor. Even if dogs cannot break into these cages, they can harass the occupants. Terrified rabbits and guinea pigs can race around in their cages and break their legs. Keep your dogs out of rooms containing floor cages. Use a barrier or a gate across the doorway if you are not certain that everyone in the family will remember to keep the doors closed.

Be Careful Where You Locate Aquariums

Some dogs pay no attention to aquariums; some are attracted to the movement of swimming fish and may try to jump up to investigate. Metal stands for large aquariums may not be sturdy enough to prevent tipping when large dogs jump against them. Water-filled aquariums are very heavy and may resist the efforts of even large dogs, but aquarium accessories such as lids, pumps, and filters may go flying when a dog leaps against the glass.

Small pets such as gerbils and reptiles are often kept in aquariums with screened tops. When dogs knock these off tables, the destruction is absolute. Not only are pets injured and lost, but shards of glass, bedding, and food are spread throughout the room. If your dogs show any interest in animals behind glass, keep them away from aquariums.

Rabbits and Ferrets

Never allow rabbits and ferrets to be loose when you are away. Rabbits can be trained to use a litter pan. So can ferrets—at least some of them can. People who keep pet rabbits and ferrets often allow them to run loose in selected rooms in their house, but if you have dogs as well as rabbits or ferrets, don't do it!

Rabbits are rather fragile creatures. One nip from a dog can tear a large piece of skin off a rabbit; one yank can break a leg. Ferrets are less easily damaged and more likely to escape the unwanted attentions

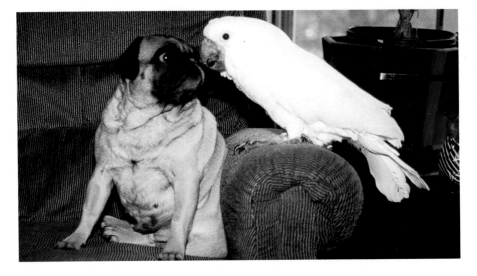

This cockatoo is unusually friendly. Many big birds will bite dogs.

of your dog, but you take a chance every time your pets are loose together. Be safe—keep them apart.

Birds

Never trust a bird to stay out of harm's way just because it can fly. Cage birds get little chance to practice their flying skills; they tire easily and often land in places that may place them within reach of your dog. Canaries, budgerigars, and birds of similar size can be crushed to death with one snap. It's fun to have your bird perch on your shoulder, but when you leave the room, put the bird back in its cage or take the dog with you.

Can Some Birds Harm Your Dog?

Owners of large psittacines such as Amazon parrots, African grays, cockatoos, and macaws know how hard these birds can bite. The bird that is perfectly friendly with people can be a menace to other animals. Psittacine birds bite not only to defend themselves; they often are very protective of their territories and jealous of their owners' attentions. Birds of the parrot family may attack dogs and other animals that come too close to their cages or their owners; so, be careful if you keep your large parrot on a perch; it may decide to jump down onto your dog or cat.

Parrotlike birds are wasteful feeders; they throw a significant amount of their food onto the bottom of the cage or onto the floor. Many dogs relish these discarded scraps of seed, shells, and fruit. If your dog scavenges under your parrot's cage, be sure it does not find enough bird food to give it indigestion.

Chapter Thirteen

Livestock, Large and Small

In the early part of the twentieth century, most of the population of the United States lived on farms, owned dogs and farm animals, and allowed the dogs to run loose. Originally, dog licenses were sold to raise money to reimburse farmers for livestock killed by dogs. Tags were attached to the dogs' collars to prove that their owners had paid the licensing fee. Later in the century, the tags were numbered to identify dogs that were killed while harassing livestock, so that the owners of the dogs could be assessed for the damages. In every state in the nation, owners of livestock still have the legal right to kill any dogs found attacking their farm animals.

Keep Your Dogs at Home

Most of us regard Fido to be as much a member of the family as a son or a daughter. Would you allow your child to roller-skate in the middle of a highway? To pull up your neighbor's rosebushes? To walk into McDonalds' and grab someone else's burger? To pick fights with local children? Of course not. If your child did these things, you would find yourself visiting a hospital or in juvenile court; yet countless dog owners open the door and let Fido run loose, confident that he will eventually come home.

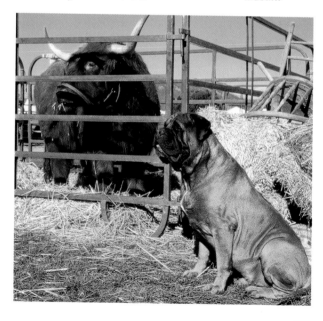

Two tough guys— Scottish Highland Bull and Bull Mastiff.

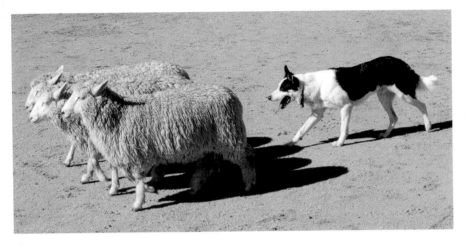

Loose dogs are struck by automobiles, attacked by other dogs, infected with diseases and parasites, lost, stolen, and impounded. Loose dogs in rural areas chase sheep, catch chickens, harass cattle, break into rabbit pens, and are captured or killed by livestock owners. Landowners need not prove that your dog is actually harassing their livestock. The presence of dogs in the vicinity of farm animals is enough to give farmers the legal right to shoot your dog. If your dog is impounded, you will have to pay a hefty fine to reclaim it, even if it is not accused of causing damage. If you value your dogs, keep them behind a fence, on a chain, or under the control of your voice.

Note. Because of dogs' social nature, loose dogs often run together in packs. In most rural areas, these packs consist of owned animals that are not confined. Obviously, two or more dogs roaming together can do many times the damage to farm animals than can one dog alone.

Sheep

Sheep seem to be born to be prey. They are described as witless, stupid animals that are easily terrified into running into fences and sustaining massive injuries. If they do not die from their injuries, they succumb to exhaustion and fright. Unfortunately, this is a good description of the domestic sheep. Two or more dogs attacking sheep often results in the death of several sheep and severe damage to the remainder of the flock.

Dogs that attack sheep are not necessarily bloodthirsty killers. Crossbred as well as purebred dogs of the collie and shepherd types inherit enough of the herding instinct to cause them to chase any animal that runs. Sheep-chasers are merely obeying this instinct. Since sheep are not large enough to appear threatening to the average farm dog, they become ideal prey. At home, the sheep-killer may be a devoted pet; at large, it is a menace.

You can train your dog to stay away from your sheep *when you are present.* Simply train it, on leash at first, where it can see your flock. Insist on obedience to *down, come,* and *heel.* Correct with the head halter and your voice any movement the dog makes toward the sheep. When it obeys in the presence of the flock, you can allow the dog freedom, but call it back at the first sign of interest in your sheep.

If your dog's chasing instinct is strong enough, you might not be able to train it to stay away from your sheep when you are not in sight. You probably will not be able to train it to stay away from your neighbor's sheep, or even your own sheep if they are in a different pasture. Protect your sheep: Install fences of woven wire that reach clear to the ground so dogs cannot run under the fence. Keep your dogs confined or in your sight when your sheep are on pasture.

Poultry

Anything with feathers is a natural prey species to a dog, even if it is a domestic bird. If your dog has any hunting instinct at all, you will not train it not to chase and kill loose poultry in your yard. The most you

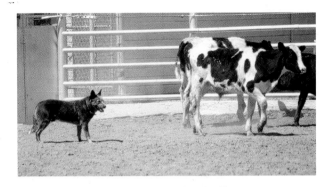

can hope for is to train your dog well enough to be able to call it back from its chase.

Large geese and swans have been known to intimidate dogs, but the dog driven away by an aggressive gander will still take its chances with a Pekin duck. Keep your poultry behind fences strong enough to resist dogs' claws. If you have a problem with stray dogs, common chicken wire should be reinforced at the bottom.

The Australian Cattle Dog can work cattle, sheep, and goats with skill.

Cattle

Cattle are often aggressive toward other animals, and will stand their ground when dogs approach. Cattle with horns may use them against dogs; cattle without horns still defend themselves with their massive foreheads. Cattle of all types are quite agile at kicking dogs.

It is not likely that one dog alone will harm mature cattle, although a pack of dogs can do significant damage to calves.

Chapter Fourteen
Dogs and Horses

This Labrador Retriever is completely safe around horses.

Before the twentieth century, horses and mules supplied the power for transportation and land cultivation in the United States. Until the automobile and the tractor gradually supplanted the need for horsepower, 20 million horses were at work in the nation. The United States now has a horse population of about 12 million, nearly all of which are used in equine sports, racing, and personal recreation. A few cattle ranchers and members of some religious groups still depend on horses to herd their stock, pull their buggies, and till their fields.

Horses and dogs have existed together since the horse was domesticated. Mounted riders hunt with packs of hounds. Guard dogs are kept in stables to discourage theft, eliminate rats, and warn of intruders. Dalmatian dogs are traditional followers of horse-drawn carriages. Trail riders, both children and adults, enjoy having their dogs accompany them on their excursions; yet dogs and horses are very different animals. The ancestors of *Canis familiaris,* the domestic dog, were predators that killed other animals for survival. The ancestors of *Equus caballas,* the domestic horse, were prey species that often were killed by packs of canines. Conflict is always possible when the modern versions of these two ancient species get together.

Horse-proof Your Dogs

Even the smallest pony is bigger than all but the largest dog. Horses are instinctively wary of dogs and all animals that might be prey species.

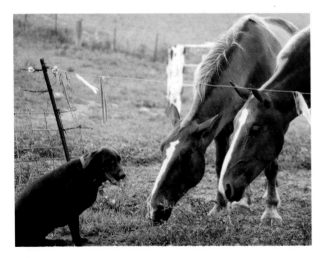

The horse's first line of defense is to run away; dogs can chase horses into fences and cause them serious harm.

Horses can hurt dogs on purpose. The horse's second line of defense is to strike, kick, or bite its attackers. Many horses have learned to launch vicious attacks at dogs that approach them.

Horses can hurt dogs by accident. A dog may be killed or maimed if it gets underfoot and is stepped on by a horse. If your dogs are to be safe around horses, they must never threaten a horse, never chase a horse, and never get too close to a horse's hooves. To keep your dog safe from horses, it must learn never to approach a horse close enough to be kicked or stepped on.

Introducing Your Dog to Horses

The younger the dog, the easier it will be to train it to be safe around horses. Start as soon as your pup has learned to walk on a leash.

- Walk your pup through the stable when the horses are in their stalls. Tell it *"No! No!"* and pull it away when it tries to approach the stalls to investigate. Keep your puppy at least 3 feet (91 cm) away from the stalls and offer it praise and a treat when it ignores the horses.
- Walk back and forth through the stable, repeating the lesson, for ten minutes once or twice a day. Your puppy will learn never to get too close to horses and to pay attention only to you. Neither les-

At no time should you ever allow your puppy or dog to approach horses to "make friends" or to "learn that horses are harmless." Horses are not harmless to dogs. Horses are easily startled into kicking a dog and large enough to step on a dog unintentionally. Never think that "one little kick" will teach a dog to beware of horses. One little kick may be enough to kill your dog.

son will be difficult. A young dog will be suspicious of unfamiliar huge animals, and the treat in your hand will keep its attention focused on yourself.

- Take the leash off when your puppy consistently ignores the horses. If it approaches the stalls closer than it should, tell it *"No! No!"* while you turn and briskly walk away. When it starts to follow you, tell it *"Come"* and offer the treat. Praise it when it complies. If it does not respond correctly, put the leash back on for a few more lessons. Use a startle device (water pistol, soda can full of pebbles or coins, air horn) to frighten your puppy if it persists in getting close to the horses.
- If the dog is an adult when you teach it safety around horses, start with the same technique as for a puppy. Walk it, on leash, through the stable; reprimand it when it tries to approach the horses; reward it when its attention stays focused on

you. After a lesson or two, start to practice *heel, down,* and *come* in the stable instead of just walking back and forth. If your dog is still young or apt to disobey off leash, keep the leash on until it is under control with the leash removed.

• Once your dog obeys in the presence of horses in their stalls, repeat the lesson with horses loose in a paddock or being led or ridden nearby. Keep the dog on a leash. At first, try to keep the horses to a walk as running horses will encourage the dog to give chase. Allow the horses to trot only when the dog obeys *heel* and *down* while the horses walk. Every time the dog makes a move toward a horse, call it away.

All dogs are different. If you have a puppy of a breed not designed for herding, hunting, or guarding, it should learn to stay away from horses with a few days' lessons. If you have an adult dog of a herding breed that instinctively wants to chase other animals, it may take weeks. It will take even longer if your dog has not been taught to obey in the presence of all distractions. A few dogs can never be trained to be safe around horses. If yours is one of these, keep it on a chain.

When to Allow Your Dog Freedom

Release the dog from your voice commands or leash and allow it to run loose only when you have seen that it will obey consistently in the presence of horses, even trotting or galloping horses. Both adult dogs and puppies should be willing to come to you (for praise and/or a treat) while horses are running in the pasture or being ridden past. If your dog shows any inclination to chase, it should still be on a leash. It should stay on a leash or a long rope until you are sure of its actions.

Breeds of dogs such as Border Collies instinctively herd livestock by nipping at their heels and dodging their kicks. These breeds are very trainable and can be trusted when their handlers are present. The instinct to herd is so strong in some members of these breeds that they can never be trusted around loose horses in the absence of their handlers. They will always try to herd livestock and will always be at risk of causing damage to the stock or to themselves.

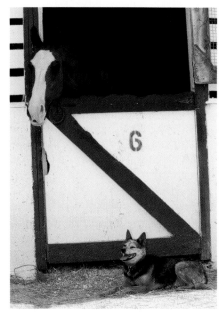

"Down-stay" in the stable.

Training Your Dog to Follow You on Horseback

Trail riders often enjoy taking their dogs along with them. If you would like your dog to accompany you on your riding excursions, be sure the dog will come home safely with you.

- Only take your dog along if it will keep away from horses' hooves.
- Only take your dog if it will stay with you and come when you call. Wandering dogs become lost or injured. A dog that will dependably stay with its owner on foot will stay with its owner on horseback.
- Take your dog only if it is physically able to keep up with you on horseback and to travel as far as you will ride. If you like to race other riders, it is best to leave your dog at home; no dog can keep up for long with galloping horses.
- If your route includes crossing paved roads, take your dog along only if it will stay behind your horse

and not dash ahead into traffic. Cars kill far more dogs than horses do.

The very small dog, the old dog, almost any dog in extremely hot weather—these are the ones that should wait at the stable for your return. A dog that cannot keep up may be lost before a rider notices its absence. In hot weather, a dog may run itself into a heat stroke while a horse is traveling at a gentle trot.

Training Your Dog to Heel Behind Your Horse

If your travels on horseback will take you across paved roads or into traffic, train your dog to heel behind your horse. This is surprisingly easy to do once your dog has learned to heel off leash when you are on foot. If it has not, train it to heel correctly before you teach it to heel when you are on horseback.

Your dog should not heel right at the horse's left hind leg; that position

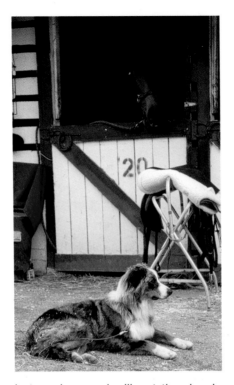

Australian Shepherds are popular among horse owners.

is too close and will put the dog in danger if the horse takes a sudden step sideways. The correct position for a dog heeling with a horse is 2 or 3 feet (61–91 cm) behind and to the left of the horse.

Presuming that your dog obeys the *heel* command off leash and in every situation, here is how you train it to heel next to your horse:

1. Get a friend to ride the horse at a walk. Your dog should be well enough trained to heel off leash. With your dog at heel, walk behind the horse and 3 feet away from the horse's left hip.

2. Ask your rider friend to change directions, to stop and start. Follow the horse, stopping when it

does. Your dog should sit when you stop. Enforce the *heel* command with your voice and leash if the dog makes a mistake. Stay 3 feet behind and to the left side of the horse. If your dog is properly trained to heel, it will ignore the horse and obey you in only one lesson. If the dog seems confused by the presence of the horse, give it three or four ten-minute lessons at heel while you walk behind the horse.

3. Change places with your rider friend. Now you are mounted and the friend is walking 3 feet behind the horse's left hip with your dog at heel. If your dog seems reluctant to obey the commands of a stranger, have your friend keep it on a leash for the first few minutes. Ask your friend to give the *heel* command only the very first time you urge the horse to walk. Give every subsequent command yourself, and speak loudly enough for your dog to hear you over the sound of the horses' hooves.

4. Practice this for ten minutes. You are mounted. You are giving all the commands. Your friend is walking next to the horse's hip with the dog at heel. Whenever you stop the horse, your friend stops and the dog sits. You command the dog "*Jack, heel*" whenever you start the horse. Your friend starts to walk whenever the horse walks, stops whenever the horse stops, but says nothing to the dog.

5. Ask your friend to go sit in the shade and watch the dog do it by itself. It is that easy. Your dog will heel behind and to the left of the horse that you are riding just as if you or your friend were still walking there. Virtually every dog that is dependable at heel will perform well, although some dogs will require repeated voice commands from the rider.

6. Ask your dog to heel behind the horse whenever it could get into trouble if it were loose. Release it from the position by the same command you use to release it from the *heel* position when you are on foot: *"Okay, Jack."* At the next crossroad, call it back into the heel position: *"Jack, heel."*

A dog should not be asked to heel for long next to a trotting horse, although a slow jog for limited periods of time can be used to increase a dog's stamina. A dog should never be permitted to heel next to a horse at a canter or gallop; these gaits are too fast for a dog to follow at heel.

Never expect a dog heeling next to a horse to maintain as accurate a position as it would when heeling next to a person. This is not an obedience trial exercise. Be willing to accept any position behind the horse's left hip, and do not insist on *sit* when you stop the horse. The dog may be too cautious to be willing to sit near a horse's hooves.

If your dog is not perfect the first time, go back to step 3 for another lesson or two. If it still is not perfect, it needs more training at heel with the handler on foot.

If you want two or more dogs to accompany you on your rides, train each of them individually to heel behind the horse, then work them together. With several dogs, you may need a walking helper at first.

Training Your Dog to Follow a Horse-drawn Vehicle

It is less difficult to train a dog to stay behind a carriage than to heel next to a mounted horse, because the trainer gets to ride; someone else drives the horse while the trainer sits at the back of the vehicle and instructs the dog on a leash. Once the dog understands, the leash is removed. An interesting reference for this procedure is included in Useful Addresses and Literature, beginning on page 134.

Dog-proof Your Horse

Your horse does not see the world as you do. Horses' vision is not like humans' vision because horses' eyes are more nearly on the sides of their heads than are human's eyes; therefore, they see most things with one eye at a time. Unlike humans, horses have no close-up binocular (with both eyes) vision at all. They can only see objects directly in front of them that are at a distance. A horse has no need to see the grain it is eating nor the grass it is grazing; it uses its nose and lips to identify its food.

Because of the location of their eyes, horses have excellent vision to the side, and fair vision behind them. Horses are very quick to notice movement in their visual fields. Their wild ancestors escaped death because they could detect predators approaching from all directions.

Keeping all that in mind, unless your horse is accustomed to the presence of dogs, it may be startled into running or kicking whenever a dog comes near. Your horse's panic reaction can cause serious harm to humans as well as to the horse itself.

When you trained your dog to stay at least 3 feet (91 cm) away from horses' hooves, you were allowing your horse to see that the presence of a dog was not a threat. When you enforced your dog's correct behavior in the presence of a horse being led or ridden, you were also teaching the horse that the dog would not come any closer. Even foals will soon learn to ignore a dog that it is being trained in the isle of the stable or outside the paddock or pasture fence.

When your dog could be trusted at liberty in the presence of horses, your horse discovered that even loose dogs are not going to attack, but what if stray dogs chase your horse? Will the horse be at increased risk because it is not afraid?

Your horse will actually be safer than one that is terrified of dogs. The horse that flees in panic from a dog is the one that runs into fences and other objects that cause it to be injured. The horse that is accustomed to dogs is the one that will stand and fight by kicking or striking at stray dogs.

Yes, if your horse is not afraid of dogs, attacking dogs will be at increased risk. Eliminate a nuisance: Inform your neighbors that your horses will harm their dogs. They will then keep their dogs at home!

Training Your Horses to Like Dogs

Take your dog to the stable with you at feeding time. If the dog is trained, have it sit or lie down nearby in the isle while you give each horse its grain ration. Your horses will learn to associate the presence of the dog with something good—the arrival of the grain. If your dog is not yet dependable on *sit* or *down,* tie your dog in the isle while you give the horses their grain. There is no harm if the tied dog jumps around and barks; the horses will learn to ignore it in anticipation of their meal.

Under no circumstances should you *ever* permit your dog to enter a horse's stall, with you or without you. A dog confined in a small area with a horse is in danger; the horse may hurt the dog accidentally or intentionally. A horse can be as protective of its territory and its feed as can a dog. Reinforce the lesson by never allowing a dog to enter a stall even when the horse is not in it. Horses' stalls should be off-limits at all times!

Dogs That Are Frightening to Horses

Horses are more likely to be startled by large and light-colored dogs because large, light dogs and white-spotted dogs are much more notice-able than are small dark ones. If you own only a Schipperke, consider inviting a friend who owns a Great Pyrenees to visit so your horses can see that not all dogs are small and black. If this is impractical, you might have your Skip occasionally wear a white sweater (or pin a white towel around it) to acquaint your horses with dogs of light colors.

Horseback Riders

Horseback riders who travel public roads or even park trails are often confronted with the menace of loose dogs. Most such incidents are innocuous, but some may end in disaster to the horse and rider.

Never take a chance of losing control of your horse. The faster a horse is moving, the more difficult it is to control it. A novice rider has a good chance of handling a horse at a walk, but a horse at a gallop can tax the ability of an expert. If you are bucked off, you might be injured and your horse might run into traffic. Whenever you get in trouble on a horse, never try to run away from it. *Slow down!*

If you ride past farmhouses, you may be accosted by farm dogs that dash out onto the road. These dogs chase riders for the same reason that they chase cars: to drive intrud-ers away from their property. Few of these "guard" dogs will chase a horse (or a car) beyond the bound-aries of their yards. If a farm dog runs out as you ride by, continue past the property at a walk or slow trot. If you urge your horse into a gallop, the dog may terrify your horse by chasing farther and barking louder. A frightened horse will try to run or try to buck, either of which may result in disaster.

A rider in a public park is seldom bothered by a single loose dog unless the rider permits the horse to run away, which may encourage the dog to chase; however, packs of loose dogs in a public park take courage from one another and may pursue a horse and rider.

If you cannot walk your horse away from stray dogs, turn to face them. If you have enough control of your mount, advance toward the pack at a walk. Because of its size, most dogs will be intimidated when a horse comes toward them.

If you are afraid of losing control of your horse, use one rein to keep it turning in small circles. A horse that is turning cannot bolt away with you. If you are afraid that your horse will rear, urge it forward; if you think it will buck, don't let it get its head down.

Chapter Fifteen

Dogs at Large

Not every dog *owner* is a dog *lover*. The thousands of dogs roaming the public streets and parks of every city attest to this fact. Owners who love their dogs would never allow them to run loose to be lost, stolen, killed by cars, and attacked by other dogs.

Dogs running at large are a threat to dogs whose owners keep them under proper restraint. In some communities, the problem is so severe that owners hesitate to exercise their dogs in their own yards because they fear an attack by a pack of strays. What can you do to protect yourself and your dogs from this menace?

How to Protect Yourself and Your Dogs from Strays

- *Call the dog warden.* In most communities, this is probably a waste of time. Animal control officers in the larger cities may try to capture strays, but their primary function is to impound unwanted animals and to enforce leash laws, not to chase loose dogs all over town. The owners, if any, of the majority of dogs running loose are unknown; however, if you happen to know who owns the dogs, the officers can issue citations and can impound the dogs of repeat offenders.
- *Stay out of the most dangerous areas.* Walk your dog only in places in which strays do not congregate. Unfortunately, loose dogs are most common in the nicest areas for dog-walking: parks and open spaces.
- *Be extra cautious when you see more than one loose dog.* Dogs instinctively hunt in packs. Two or more dogs running together are far more dangerous than a single dog. A pack of loose dogs may establish a territory, just as a gang of teenagers may establish a territory of a few city blocks. If you and your dog enter the dogs' territory, you may be subject to harassment and injury.

- *Keep your own dog on a leash.* Even though your dog may be well trained, keep it close to you. A dog is more subject to attack by strays if it is at a distance from a human.

Dealing with Loose Dogs

Loose and stray dogs are not friendly. They avoid contact with people. Strays are usually large breeds, mixed breeds, not neutered, not trained, and carriers of parasites. If a loose dog seeks human contact, however, it actually may be someone's lost pet. Examine it for a collar and tag; you may be able to help it get home.

Attacks by Loose Dogs

In almost every case, attacks by loose dogs are directed toward the leashed dog, not the owner, but few owners will drop the leash and abandon their dogs to their fate. Owners who attempt to break up dogfights risk being bitten on purpose by the strange dogs and by accident by their own dogs defending themselves.

To prevent attacks from starting, take immediate action when loose dogs appear. Walk, do not run, out of the areas as quickly as you can. Try to prevent your own dog from barking or growling, which will attract the attention of the strays.

If you have a very small dog, pick it up and cover it with your coat so the strays do not recognize it as possible prey. If you cannot hide your dog with your coat, consider not picking it up. You will be at increased risk of being bitten yourself if the strays jump up to attack a dog in your arms.

If the strays follow you, enter a building, a car, or a park shelter as quickly as possible. Stay inside until the strays lose interest and leave.

Carry a Weapon

People approached by strange dogs are advised to stand still and keep quiet. These rules do not apply when you have a dog with you, since your dog will neither stand still nor be quiet. If there may be strays where you walk your dog, carry something to protect yourself and your dog.

A canister of pepper spray, properly directed, will deter attacking dogs but the problem is to get the canister out of your pocket and direct the spray only toward the attackers while your own dog is leaping around at the end of its leash. A noisemaker, such as a foghorn or a battery-operated ultrasonic training device, will probably be effective against most attacks. A few dogs will ignore devices that produce only noise in the range of ultrasound.

If you are hesitant about handling pepper sprays and question the efficacy of noisemakers, you still need a weapon that is easy to carry and frightening to stray dogs. One object that meets these criteria is a large umbrella.

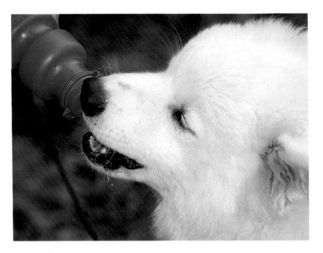

The Samoyed enjoys a drink after jogging with its owner.

A man's umbrella can be carried rolled up as a cane and it can be opened quickly. Although it is made of thin fabric, an umbrella looks like a large, impressive barrier when thrust toward a dog. If a dog tears the fabric, you still will have the handle and the metal ribs to use as a weapon.

If you prefer to carry a smaller object, get a collapsible, telescoping umbrella that shoots open when you press a button on the handle. This type of umbrella is usually less than 16 inches (41 cm) long and has a wrist loop. Choose a man's umbrella, which is larger than a lady's umbrella; choose a black one, which is more threatening to a dog than a light-colored one. Buy a cheap umbrella in case it is destroyed. Carry the umbrella with its covering case removed, so that you can open it in a hurry.

Separating the Fighters

If you see one or more stray dogs in the area, get your defenses ready before you need them. If you cannot escape the dogs' approach, turn to face them and use your spray or your noisemaker. If you have an umbrella, open it and shove it between the strays and yourself. Keep your own dog close to your legs.

If your dog actually is attacked, do not hesitate to use pepper spray to break up the fight. Your own dog will be sprayed too, but it will recover more easily from a dose of pepper than from severe bite wounds. If you have an umbrella, open it and jab the point at the attacking dog. Be cautious about kicking and yelling at fighting dogs; one of them might turn and grab your leg.

Jogging with Your Dog

Jogging with a dog is very popular in the city. The jogger has company and the dog, as well as the owner, gets exercise; however, jogging with your dog may be good for your health, but may not be good for the health of your dog.

Dedicated joggers cover many miles in all kinds of weather. They usually jog on pavement or public roadways. They dress in layers of clothing that they can vary according to the weather and wear shoes appropriate to the terrain. As their condition improves, joggers increase the speed and distance of their daily jogs.

When a jogger takes a dog along, the dog has no choice but to travel the same terrain for the same distance and at the same speed as does its owner, but a dog must jog barefoot on every kind of pavement. A dog jogs on the same pads on ice as it does on hot asphalt.

A dog cannot add or remove clothing if it gets cold or overheated. A dog can only pant to dissipate its body heat; it cannot sweat. Panting is far less effective in cooling a body than is sweating, so dogs are easily jogged into dangerously high body temperatures. Remember these important points:

- Before you take your dog jogging, be sure it is able to tolerate as much exercise as you are.
- Be sure that the road conditions will not be harmful to its feet.
- If you take bottled water to quench your thirst, take some sort of container from which you can also offer water to your dog. *Never* rely on finding a possibly contaminated puddle from which it can get a drink.
- If your dog pants heavily or starts to lag behind, stop and walk until its breathing is normal.
- If you have an older dog, a small dog, or a heavily coated dog, you may want to leave it home and jog alone.

Jogging and Strays

Jogging is faster than walking, and may excite stray dogs into pursuit. If you are approached by loose dogs, stop and stand still. Never appear to be running away. Turn to face the dogs. Use your pepper spray, your horn, or your umbrella if necessary,

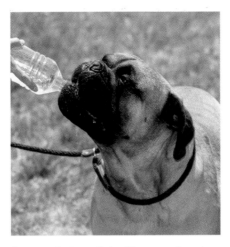

This Bull Mastiff shares its owner's bottled water.

then walk to safety. Resume jogging only when there is no danger that the loose dogs will chase you.

Bicycling with Your Dog

Bicycling with a dog is never a good idea. Bicycling is always done on hard pavement, often in dangerous traffic. The leash can become tangled in the spokes or bicycle chain, causing a nasty spill and an injured dog and/or rider. Bicycling with your dog off leash is a *very* bad idea; the dog can become separated from you and struck by a car. Your dog can be easily exhausted running next to your bicycle, even though you might not notice the strain.

Bicycling and Strays

Loose dogs are very likely to chase bicycles; dogs accompanying bicycles make ready victims. If you insist on taking your dog along when you ride your bicycle, keep alert for strays. Stop and get off the bicycle *before* you and your dog are attacked. Keep your pepper spray handy. Walk your dog and your bicycle to safety. The only thing in favor of a riding a bicycle to exercise your dog is that a light bicycle is a handy weapon to jam between fighting dogs. You may be able to break up a fight, but your expensive 10-speed may sustain as much damage as does your dog.

Bite Wounds

There is no way of knowing if a stray dog has been vaccinated against rabies. Dog bite wounds are often deep punctures and contaminated with dirt. If you or your dog is bitten by a stray, seek immediate medical care.

If the biting dog can be captured, it should be impounded and examined for rabies. In most cases, the biting dog escapes. The owner of the bitten dog, a veterinarian, and a physician (if the owner has also been bitten) must decide an appropriate course of medical treatment.

When Your Dog Is Bitten by a Stray

• Have your dog's wounds treated as soon as possible. If it is bleeding profusely, has large areas of torn skin, or seems to have difficulty breathing, rush your dog to the nearest veterinary hospital or animal emergency clinic. If its

injuries appear to be less serious, take it to your own veterinarian that same day.
• Your dog should receive a rabies vaccine immediately unless it has had a rabies booster within the last six months. If your dog has had the booster, your veterinarian may consider its protection to be satisfactory. Rabies is one of the few diseases for which a vaccine given after the exposure is effective.
• The attending veterinarian may prescribe antibiotics to prevent the dog's wounds from becoming infected. The veterinarian may also prescribe medication for you to apply to the dog's wounds. Be sure to use the medication for as long as indicated, even if the dog seems to have recovered before the medicine is gone.
• Tetanus (lockjaw) is relatively uncommon in dogs. Dog bite wounds are often punctures, which increase the possibility of this disease. The veterinarian will decide if tetanus *antitoxin* (serum containing antibodies against the disease) should be given to your dog.

If You Are Bitten by a Stray

• Your wounds should be treated immediately. If you cannot reach your own physician, go to a hospital emergency room.
• If the biting dog can be captured, it can be quarantined for ten days under veterinary supervision. Dogs showing no signs of rabies within ten days are considered not to have been able to transmit rabies

to humans or other animals at the time of the bite.

- If the biting dog is captured, it can be killed and its brain examined for the presence of microscopic structures, *fluorescent antibodies,* that indicate rabies. The brain of the biting dog must not be damaged in order for this test to be performed. The brain of a dog killed by shooting or clubbing it on the head will be useless for examination.
- If the biting dog cannot be captured and examined for rabies, you may be advised to undergo rabies preventive treatment. The new methods of treating people who might have been exposed to rabies are less painful than the older methods, but they are quite expensive. If rabies is common in your locality, your physician and the local health official will certainly recommend the treatment.

Rabies is spread only when the infectious saliva of a rabid animal enters the broken skin or mucous membranes of another animal. The fact that you were in the presence of an animal that *might* have been rabid does not mean that you were necessarily exposed; however, once the signs of rabies develop in a person, the disease is invariably fatal. Your physician will help you decide whether to undergo treatment.

- Ask your doctor if you need an injection against tetanus. Humans are more susceptible to tetanus than are dogs. If you have not had a tetanus vaccine within the last three years, your physician may recommend that you receive a tetanus *antitoxin*. If your tetanus protection is up to date, your doctor may administer a tetanus *toxoid,* which acts as a booster shot for your immunity.
- The attending physician will decide if you need antibiotics, and will prescribe medication for your wounds. Take everything as directed.

If Strays Get into Your Own Yard

Even if your dogs are safely confined behind a fence, loose dogs can be a danger to them. Few loose dogs will attempt to climb or jump into a fenced area, unless the area contains a bitch in heat. A strong, high fence will prevent loose dogs from attacking yours, but your dog is almost certain to defend its boundaries by running along the fence and snarling viciously. If the loose dogs come near enough, your dog may injure its mouth and break its teeth when it attacks the wire fence.

If you live in an area where loose dogs are common, consider one of these methods to protect your dog:

- Install a strong fence, at least 4 feet (122 cm) high, depending on the size of your dog. Do not use chicken wire and do not install low fences, even if you have toy breeds. Most loose dogs will not jump into another dog's yard unless the fence is less than 3 feet (91 cm) high.

- Use wire fence with openings of 2 inches (5 cm) or less. The smaller the openings between the wires, the safer and sturdier the fence will be. Dogs can get their teeth through 3-inch (7.6 cm) openings.
- Keep bitches in heat indoors when they are not supervised.
- Install the fence close to the ground; bury the bottom of the fence, or place a barrier such as rocks, logs, or sod at the bottom of the fence. This will prevent your dog from digging under the fence.
- Consider using palisade or solid board fencing to prevent fence-fighting. Do not use plastic strips woven into chain-link fencing. These are soon torn out by active dogs.
- Do not expect electronic boundaries to protect your dogs from strays. Electronic containment systems such as the "Invisible Fence" affect only dogs wearing receiver collars. Your dog may be trapped within its own yard if it will not cross the boundary line.
- Do not leave an unattended dog chained in your yard without a means of escape. It will be at the mercy of wandering strays. A doghouse for it to run into may not be adequate protection.

Avoid tragedies and lawsuits! If you are the owner of a dog with a strong predatory or territorial instinct, be sure that it cannot escape your control and attack other dogs or children.

If Your Dog Is an Offender

You know the nature of your own dog. You know if your dog has demonstrated the tendency to attack smaller animals as if they were prey or to challenge strange dogs on the street. You know if you must exercise extreme caution to prevent your dog from escaping your control.

If your dog gets off your property and attacks another dog, you might have to pay expensive veterinary bills for the other dog's owner. You might even have to buy your neighbor another dog. Your dog could be quarantined for rabies or declared a dangerous animal.

If your dog leaves your yard and attacks a child, or a person walking a dog, you will be the defendant in a lawsuit. You will have huge legal expenses and court appearances. You will have to pay fines and damages. You will have to live with the guilt caused by your carelessness. The court may order your dog to be euthanized.

Never take chances. Train your dog not to rush past you whenever you open a door. Install high fences and check them often for damage. Look at the bottom of the fence to see if your dog is trying to dig under. Install locks on all the gates and keep them locked. If you chain your dog, examine your chain for weak snaps and worn links. Be sure that your dog cannot escape and cause irreparable harm to innocent animals or people.

Chapter Sixteen

Viral and Bacterial Diseases

About 100 years ago, it was not unusual for children to die of diphtheria. It was not unusual for dogs to die of canine distemper, or for cats to succumb to feline panleucopenia. Today we have vaccines against so many contagious diseases of humans and animals that only the children and pets of careless or uninformed parents or owners need suffer or die from most contagious diseases.

Viral Diseases

The majority of all viral diseases affect only one genus or only one species of animal. Such diseases are said to be *host-specific*.

Some diseases that affect different animals may have the same common name. Dog distemper, cat distemper, and horse distemper are not the same. Each of these diseases is caused by a different organism; each species cannot get distemper from the other species.

Rabies

Rabies is a viral disease from which no affected animal recovers. It can be spread from any infected mammal to every susceptible mammal of any species, including humans.

Rabies is caused by a *neurotropic* virus, one that replicates (reproduces) within the brain and nervous system of the affected animal. An animal can be infected with rabies for weeks or months before it shows abnormal behavior or other signs of the disease. The rabies virus appears in the saliva of a rabid animal only during the infectious stages of the disease. A rabid animal spreads rabies when its saliva enters a wound or a scratch on an uninfected mammal.

The rabies virus exists in wildlife populations such as skunks, raccoons, foxes, coyotes, and bats. There are at least five strains of the rabies virus in the United States; each strain is prevalent in a specific wild animal. There is evidence that every strain of the virus is able to cause rabies in most species of mammals.

Rabies is brought to pets and humans when susceptible domestic animals are bitten by rabid wild animals and return to their homes infected with the rabies virus. Infected domestic animals spread rabies when they develop the disease and bite or scratch uninfected pets or humans. Fortunately, there are ways to eliminate almost completely the threat of rabies to your animals and your family:

- *Have every one of your animals vaccinated.* Effective, safe, and inexpensive vaccines against rabies are available for almost all species of domestic mammals. All dogs and cats over three months of age, all horses, cattle, sheep, and goats should be vaccinated against rabies. The vaccine should be repeated every year or every third year, depending on the ages of the animals, the recommendations of the producers of the vaccine, and the advice of the administering veterinarians.

- *Keep your animals confined.* Never allow your dogs, cats, or other animals to run loose where they might come into contact with rabid wild animals that could infect them with the deadly rabies virus. Most wild animals are more active at night. *Always* keep your animals confined after dark.

- *Never touch a wild animal or any unknown domestic animal, particularly those that behave in an abnormal manner.* Rabid animals may act injured, tame, sleepy, or vicious. Under no circumstances

should you allow your children or pets to approach any strange animal. Advise them to keep away from bats that they find on the ground. Call the local game warden or the humane officer to remove wild or unknown animals in a safe manner. If you can place an empty cardboard box over the animal without touching it, you will help keep the animal confined until the game warden arrives. If the animal acts in any way aggressive, stay away from it!

- *Know the history of your new animals.* Buy a puppy, kitten, cat, or dog only from owners or breeders who do not allow their animals to run loose. Loose animals risk exposure to rabies. Buy only from a person who keeps the animals up to date on all vaccinations. Buy a puppy or kitten from a shelter only if it has been relinquished to the shelter before the young animals are old enough to have been running loose. Reject an animal that was captured in the wild. You can safely buy an adult dog or cat from a shelter if the animal was relinquished by its owner and has a history of vaccination. You can buy a relinquished animal that has no history of running loose, but has not been vaccinated against rabies. Have such an animal vaccinated immediately.

- *Be cautious about accepting animals that have been strays—you never know if they have been in contact with rabid wildlife. You cannot tell if stray animals have ever been vaccinated against rabies or any other disease. If you have questions about the advisability of adopting a stray dog or cat, call your local health department or dog warden. Ask if rabies is prevalent in your area. If it is, accept only animals that have not run loose, or animals that have been previously vaccinated. Rabies is too serious a disease to take a chance.

Viral Diseases That Affect Only Canines

Canine distemper is a serious viral disease of dogs, other canine species, and ferrets. This disease is characterized by respiratory, nervous, and digestive signs, and is often fatal, especially when accompanied by bacterial infections. Canine distemper is spread when a sick dog comes into contact with a healthy one. This disease does not affect cats, horses, or humans.

Canine hepatitis is caused by a canine adenovirus that has an affinity for liver cells. Human hepatitis and canine hepatitis are not the same disease and are not spread between the species.

Parainfluenza is a respiratory virus that affects only canines.

Parvovirus and **coronavirus** affect the digestive systems of their canine victims. Parvovirus is usually much more severe than coronavirus, although both can kill. These diseases are characterized by severe

bloody diarrhea, dehydration, and sudden death.

Canine Diseases That Are Caused by Bacteria and Viruses

Kennel cough refers to a group of diseases caused by bacteria and viruses that infect the respiratory systems of dogs. *Bordetella bronchiseptica* and the *parainfluenza virus* are the organisms most often implicated in this disease, although other bacteria and viruses may be contributors. The disease is called "kennel cough" because it is very contagious; it is common in dogs that have recently been exposed to other dogs, such as in boarding kennels or shelters. Kennel cough affects only dogs.

Bacterial Diseases That Can Affect Dogs, Humans, and Other Animals

Lyme disease is caused by a bacterium that can affect dogs and humans. The causative agent of this disease, *Borrelia burgdorferi*, is carried by a tick that infests deer, rodents, and other wild animals. Lyme disease is spread when an infected tick bites another animal.

Lyme disease can be mild, severe, or even fatal. Fever is often the first sign that a dog is infected with Lyme disease; the development of other signs depends on the response of the host's body to the invasion of the bacterium. If detected early in the course of the infection, Lyme disease can be treated successfully with tetracyclines and other antibiotics.

Leptospirosis is caused by a bacterium that may be infective to dogs, humans, and perhaps other animals. The causative organisms are spread by contamination of food and water with the urine of an infected animal.

Modern Vaccines

Your dogs do not need to get eight or ten separate vaccines. Most vaccines are designed to protect your dog against four, five, or even six diseases at the same time. Your veterinarian will schedule the vaccines that your dog needs according to the dog's age and the prevalence of the disease in your locality.

The vaccine for rabies is not offered in combination with protection against other diseases. Animals receive rabies vaccines in a separate injection.

Chapter Seventeen
Internal Parasites

Parasites are organisms that live by feeding upon other animals. Most canine parasites are easily spread to other members of the dog family. Dogs and doglike animals can infect and be infected with certain parasites that are shared by animals other than dogs. Before you add another animal to your household, determine if it will bring unwanted parasitic diseases to the animals you already own.

Intestinal Parasites—Worms

Animals can become infected with internal parasites by several processes:
• Prenatal infection (spread from the mother to the young before birth).
• Accidental ingestion of parasitic eggs or larvae in contaminated food or water.
• Accidental ingestion of the intermediate host of a parasite (fleas).
• Deliberate ingestion of the intermediate host of a parasite (mice).
• The bite of a bloodsucking intermediate host (mosquito).

A diagnosis of intestinal worms is made by one of two methods:
1. The adult worms are occasionally passed in the host's stool. Some of these worms are visible to the owner and can be identified by a veterinarian.
2. The eggs of the worms are discovered by a veterinarian upon microscopic examination of the host's stool.

Medication administered for the purpose of eliminating intestinal worms is called a *vermifuge.* Each vermifuge is designed for the elimination of a specific parasite. The dose given to each individual animal is determined by the animal's weight and general condition. It is not safe for

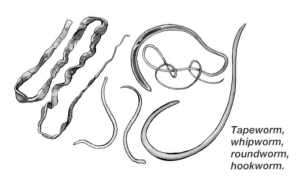

Tapeworm, whipworm, roundworm, hookworm.

Important Facts about Parasites

- An *internal parasite* is a living creature that must spend all or part of its life cycle within the body of another living animal.
- An *external parasite* must spend all or part of its life cycle feeding on or within the skin of another animal.
- A *host* is the animal within which or upon which a parasite lives.
- Some parasites are *host-specific* and can live on or within only one species of animal. Many parasites are not host-specific, and can live on or within many different families or species of hosts.
- Some parasites spend their entire lives upon or within a single host animal.
- Some parasites must occupy the bodies of more than one host or more than one species of host in order to complete their life cycles. A *final host* is the animal that harbors the adult parasite. An *intermediate host* is the animal that harbors the intermediate or larval stages of the parasite.
- Some parasites are *free-living* (not on an animal) during a portion of their lives.
- Some parasites are microscopic in size. Almost all parasite eggs are microscopic, but many adult parasites are visible to the naked eye.
- *All* parasites are harmful. Some parasites carry bacterial diseases. Many parasites in the adult or larval forms cause serious damage to the bodies of their hosts. Some may even cause the hosts' death.

owners to indiscriminately treat their animals with vermifuges. A veterinarian should recommend the correct drug, dose, and intervals of treatment for each case of intestinal worms.

Roundworms

These parasites are called roundworms because the adults are round in cross section, like the piece of spaghetti they resemble when passed in the stool of the host.

Toxocara canis and *Toxascaris leonina* are the common roundworms shared by the dog and cat. These parasites are freely exchanged between members of each species.

- An animal becomes infected with roundworms by one of two ways: It is infected before birth by roundworm larvae in its mother's tissues, or it accidentally ingests fecal material containing eggs.
- Roundworms have a direct life cycle; the adult lives in the small intestine of the host. Eggs pass from the body of the host with the feces. When the embryonated (developed) eggs are swallowed by a host, they hatch into larvae. The larvae burrow into the bloodstream of the host, migrate through the lungs, and eventually are swallowed and reach the intestines. There the

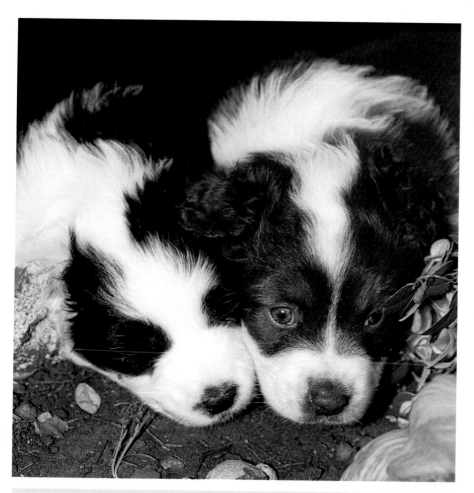

These healthy Australian Shepherd puppies are free of round-worms, but should be checked again.

Dog and Cat Roundworm May Affect Children

Visceral larval migrans is a condition that may affect humans, especially children, who accidentally get roundworm eggs on their hands and then put their hands in their mouths. Roundworm eggs ingested by humans may hatch into larvae that can migrate through other organs, and can even migrate into the chambers of the eye.

Puppies and kittens and their nursing mothers are the animals most likely to be passing roundworm eggs in their stools. Prevent infection by cleaning up stools promptly and insisting that children (and adults) always wash their hands after handling these animals.

larvae mature into adults and lay eggs.

- It is only the adult roundworms in the intestines of the host that can be eliminated by the administration of vermifuges. Some of the migrating roundworm larvae do not reach the intestines, but instead become encysted in the muscle tissue of the host. These cysts may remain in the body of the host for life.
- When a female animal that is infected with roundworms becomes pregnant, the larvae in her tissues develop into adult worms in her intestines. Treating the mother either before or during her pregnancy will not eliminate roundworm infection in her offspring. Only the mature worms in her intestines will be eliminated. The larval worms encysted in her tissues will not be destroyed. These larval worms will enter the bodies of the puppies through the placenta before the puppies are born and through her milk when the puppies nurse. *Transplacental infection* is thought not to occur in kittens. Kittens are infected with roundworms primarily through receiving the worms with their mother's milk.

Hookworms

Ancylostoma caninum and *A. brasiliense* are the common hookworms of the dog and cat. Adult hookworms are almost too small to be visible without a magnifying glass.

- Adult hookworms are attached to the lining of the host's small intestine. They feed upon blood and mucosal cells. Heavy infestation

---

Important Facts about Roundworms

- They can be spread between dogs and dogs, dogs and cats, and cats and cats.
- The stools of all new pets should be examined for the presence of the microscopic roundworm eggs. Animals that have negative stools should be checked again, just to be sure.
- Animals with positive stools should receive worm medication as directed by the veterinarian. Their stools should be checked periodically to assure that the intestinal infection is eliminated.
- Mature animals may not have roundworms in their intestines, but may have larval roundworms in their tissues. These larval worms will become adult worms in the intestines of most pregnant dogs and cats *and* their puppies and kittens.
- Most nursing dogs and cats and their offspring will pass thousands of roundworm eggs in their feces.
- All nursing dogs and cats, and their puppies and kittens should be treated with drugs at appropriate intervals to eliminate adult roundworms.

with hookworms can cause the host to become anemic from blood loss. Puppies and kittens can die from hookworm-caused anemia.

- Adult hookworms mate and lay eggs in the host animal's intestines. The eggs are passed with the feces and hatch into larvae that live and develop in the soil. Hookworm larvae molt several times before they enter the infective stage. They can live for months in the soil, awaiting a host.
- Infective hookworm larvae can be ingested accidentally or can penetrate the skin of a suitable host. Eventually the larvae migrate to the small intestine of their host and become adults, thereby completing their life cycle.
- Infective hookworm larvae cannot continue their development in a host foreign to their species. If accidentally swallowed by a human, dog and cat hookworm larvae will not develop. If they penetrate the skin of humans, the larvae of *A. brasiliense* can cause a skin rash called *cutaneous larval migrans*, but these larvae cannot develop into intestinal hookworms.
- Humans have two species of hookworm of their own, *Ancylostoma duodenale* and *Necator americanus.* Human hookworms do not infect dogs or cats.

Strongyloides **worms** of horses are related to hookworms and are similar in their life cycle. The strongyles of horses do not infect humans, dogs, or cats, although the eggs of this parasite are often found during microscopic examination of the stools of dogs that eat horse manure.

Tapeworms

All tapeworms must occupy two different hosts in order to complete their life cycles. Dogs and cats share tapeworms when they share the intermediate hosts.

The two most common tapeworms shared by dogs and cats are *Diplydium caninum,* the intermediate host of which is the flea, and *Taenia taeniaformis*, the intermediate host of which is the mouse. The life cycles of both species of tapeworms are similar.

- Tapeworms live attached to the lining of the host's small intestine, from which adult worms absorb nutrients. Egg-containing segments break off the ends of the worms and are passed from the rectum of the host, often on the surface of the bowel movements.

  Tapeworm segments, which are large enough to see, often can be found stuck to the hair around the anal areas of affected hosts. When recently passed, the segments wiggle; after a few hours, the segments dry up and resemble grains of rice. A microscopic examination of the stools of animals infected with tapeworm may not show the eggs of the worm because the eggs are contained in the segments and are not disbursed in the feces.
- When the intermediate hosts—fleas or mice—eat the tapeworm segments, they become infected with the larval stages of the tapeworm.

- Dogs and cats often swallow fleas when they lick themselves. If the fleas contain larval tapeworm, the dog or cat becomes infected with this parasite. There have been reports of humans being infected with *D. caninum* from accidentally swallowing fleas.
- Dogs and cats that catch and eat mice that contain larval tapeworms also become infected.

Neither dogs nor cats can become infected with tapeworms directly from another infected animal. Transmission requires the presence of the intermediate host. The obvious way to prevent tapeworm infection in all species is to eliminate the intermediate hosts: Eliminate fleas and keep your pets from eating mice.

Whipworms

A whipworm is actually shaped like an old-fashioned stock whip. The very thin front portion and thick rear portion of this parasite gives it its name. Adult whipworms can be more than 1 inch (2.5 cm) long but are usually not seen in dogs' stools because they are almost as thin as a hair.

Trichuris vulpis, the common dog whipworm, has a direct life cycle in which the eggs are passed in the dog's stool and develop on the ground. A dog becomes infected with whipworm by ingesting infective eggs with contaminated food, water, or soil. The egg becomes a larva in the dog's intestines. Whipworm larvae develop into adults in a portion of the dog's large intestine. A heavy infection with this parasite can result in chronic diarrhea, weight loss, and anemia in dogs.

Other species of whipworm infest cattle, swine, and even humans. These species do not live in dogs, nor do dog whipworms live in other species.

Heartworms

Of all the parasites of domestic animals, heartworm is among the most dangerous to the host. Adult heartworms, which can be up to 10 inches (25 cm) in length, live in the chambers of the host's heart and large blood vessels. These parasites disrupt normal heart action and blood circulation. The first signs of infection are exercise intolerance and a harsh cough. Severely affected animals die of circulatory failure.

Heartworm is now found almost everywhere in the continental United States. Once considered to be a parasite only of dogs, heartworm disease has been found to affect cats and other carnivores such as foxes and wolves.

- Adult worms in the heart and blood vessels produce microscopic larvae called *microfilaria.* The microfilaria circulate throughout the bloodstream of the host.
- Mosquitoes are the intermediate host of *Dirofilaria immitis,* the dog and cat heartworm. When a mosquito feeds on the blood of an infected animal, it draws the microfilaria into its body along with the blood of its victim. The microfilaria become infective in the salivary glands of the mosquito. The

Internal Parasites Transmissible among Species

Parasite	Transmissible to:		
	Dogs	*Cats*	*Others*
Roundworm	yes	yes	children
Hookworm	yes	yes	no
Tapeworm	yes	yes	humans
Whipworm	yes	no	no
Heartworm	yes	yes	carnivores
Coccidia	yes	yes	no

microfilaria gain entrance into a new host when the mosquito feeds upon an uninfected animal. Microfilaria from either dogs or cats can infect animals of the other species.

- Many animals harbor heartworm but do not show signs of the disease. It may be months or years from the time of infection before the host develops circulatory failure. If heartworm infection is diagnosed in a dog that is not yet sick, the disease can be treated successfully; once the signs are apparent, treatment is very risky.
- Heartworm infection is diagnosed by a blood test. The disease is treated by first administering a drug to kill the adult worms, later another drug to eliminate the microfilaria.
- Heartworm can be prevented much more safely and inexpensively than it can be treated. Every dog should be protected from heartworm with preventive medication. Modern heartworm preventives also help eliminate certain intestinal parasites, and need be administered only once a month.

Coccidia

Coccidia are common parasites that live in their hosts' intestines. Several species of coccidia are shared by both dogs and cats. Older animals are relatively resistant to this parasite, but kittens and puppies affected with coccidiosis suffer from severe diarrhea and dehydration.

Puppies and kittens become host to coccidia by eating objects or licking their paws contaminated with immature coccidia from the feces of other infected dogs and cats. The immature coccidia, called *oocysts,* mature in the host's intestines where they produce new oocysts that are passed in the feces and can infect other hosts.

Diagnosis of coccidiosis is made by finding the oocysts in the stools of infected animals. Coccidia are eliminated by repeated doses of an appropriate medication.

Chapter Eighteen
External Parasites

Owners are more likely to be aware of their animals' external parasites than their internal ones. Everyone can see fleas scampering through a dog's hair; everyone can observe the constant scratching of an animal infested with sarcoptes mites. Many external parasites of dogs (or of any other animal) can infest other species, can cause skin problems, and can spread disease to each animal upon which the parasite can live.

Chemical Pesticides

Never use a chemical pesticide on any animal until you have read and understood every word on the package label. If in doubt, ask your veterinarian if it is safe for the species intended; for example, certain medications work well on dogs, but will kill cats.

Never make a pesticide stronger than indicated on the label. Never use more of the drug or use it more often than the label indicates. Do not take chances. You could kill your animals while you kill their parasites.

Some external parasites are visible to the naked eye, some barely visible only in a strong light, and some can be found only when skin scrapings are examined under a microscope.

Some external parasites jump or run through the host animal's hair; some external parasites remain in one place. If you find any strange creatures on your animals, capture a few and drop them into a jar with a small amount of rubbing alcohol. The alcohol will kill them and usually preserve them enough for your veterinarian to identify them and suggest a treatment.

Common External Parasites in Pet Animals

Fleas

The flea is a true insect; it undergoes a complete metamorphosis, and adult fleas have six legs. Fleas are the most common and often the most troublesome external parasite of dogs, cats, and some other animals. *None* of the many species of fleas are entirely host-specific. Although most species have a favorite host, if they cannot find their preferred animal, fleas will infest whatever warm-blooded creatures that are available.

- The most common flea on both dogs and cats is the cat flea, *Ctenocephalides felis;* it is more common than the dog flea, *C. canis.* If any of your furred pets have fleas, the others will soon become infested.
- In the absence of dogs and cats, the *Ctenocephalides* fleas will bite humans. These fleas prefer the tender skin of children and women to men; often, the youngsters in the household are the ones with red, itchy flea bites on their legs and arms.
- The human flea, *Pulex irritans,* lives by choice on people but will also infest dogs, cats and other animals.
- Adult fleas live on the host animal, sucking blood for nourishment. It is the host's allergic reaction to the saliva of the flea that causes intense itching. Some animals seem to be more troubled by fleas than others. Even though all the animals have the same degree of flea infestation, some animals have a greater allergic response to flea saliva.
- Eggs laid by adult fleas fall off the host into the environment. Tiny, hairy, caterpillarlike larvae hatch from these eggs. They feed upon debris on the ground, molt several times, then form pupae. Eventually, the fleas emerge as

adults and seek a host upon which to feed. If you have flea eggs, larvae, or pupae in your house, they will become adult fleas and will infest new pets of every mammalian species you bring home.

As well as causing constant scratching and irritation to your pets, fleas are also the intermediate host of the common tapeworm of dogs and cats. When your pet licks and chews itself because it itches, it can accidentally swallow fleas and become infected with the larval form of tapeworms. For the good of all your pets, take steps to control this harmful parasite.

Ticks

Ticks are not insects, but are members of the family Arachnida, which also includes parasitic mites

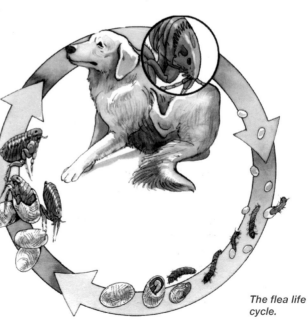

The flea life cycle.

and nonparasitic spiders and scorpions. All ticks are bloodsucking parasites of vertebrates, and can be carriers of deadly diseases such as tick paralysis, Lyme disease, and Rocky Mountain spotted fever. The bite of the tick seldom causes itching, and may not even be noticed by the host.

• Ticks in every stage of life are not host-specific. The final hosts and the intermediate hosts can be the same species or different species of animal. Most ticks prefer mammals, although some will live on birds and reptiles. In many parts of the United States, ticks infest cattle, horses, deer, and other ungulates (hoofed animals). The intermediate hosts of these ticks can be ungulates or rodents.

• Ticks have a complicated life cycle. The eight-legged adult female tick engorges on its host's blood, drops off, and lays its eggs on the ground. The eggs hatch into six-legged larvae that resemble seeds (seed ticks). These larvae crawl up blades of grass or other vegetation and wait to jump on any passing animal. The animal infested with larval ticks is called an *intermediate host.* Seed ticks gorge upon blood on an intermediate host, then again drop off onto the ground where they molt into eight-legged *nymphs.* The nymphs seek another intermediate host, feed on blood, drop off again, and molt into adults. Adult ticks jump onto *final* hosts, where they not only feed, but mate. Once their mouthparts are embedded in the skin of the host, female ticks are stationary and do not move about on the animal. Egg-bearing engorged females drop back onto the ground to lay their eggs and complete their life cycle.

• The most important ticks found on dogs are the common brown dog tick and the wood tick (*Dermacentor* sp.). An unfed brown dog tick resembles a small, fat spider. Within a few days, the adult female engorges with blood until it resembles a swollen tumor up to a ¼ inch (.5 cm) in diameter.

• If tick-infested dogs are kept in the house, female ticks will drop off the dog and lay their eggs in cracks in the floor. The eggs hatch into larvae, which are *negatively geotropic.* This means that they tend to crawl upward, away from the ground. Adult, larva, and nymph stages of ticks can be found traveling up walls and legs of furniture in search of a host. All stages of

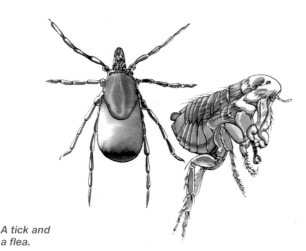

A tick and a flea.

ticks can use the same dog or dogs in the household, at different times in their cycles, as both their intermediate and final hosts.

- Since ticks will infest almost any animal, including humans, and since they can carry serious diseases, it is important to eliminate them. Even though their mouthparts are imbedded in the skin of the host, ticks should be killed with insecticide, then scraped or pulled off. Kill ticks on your dog or cat with a squirt of flea-and-tick spray that will not harm the host. Always read the label before you apply anything to your dog or cat.
- Never daub a tick with gasoline or other substance that may be harmful to skin. Never burn a tick off a living animal. The site of the removed tick should be treated with a disinfectant such as isopropyl alcohol. If mouthparts of the tick remain in the skin, they will dry up and slough away. When you remove ticks, use rubber gloves, a tissue, and tweezers or some other tool to avoid touching the tick with your hands.
- If you need the ticks for identification, drop them into a jar with a little alcohol; if not, flush them down the toilet where they cannot emerge to infest another animal.

All the ticks on an animal do not engorge at the same time. If you find even one tick, examine the animal very carefully at least once a day to find the new ones as they become engorged. Ticks' favorite places on dogs are inside the ears, on the face,

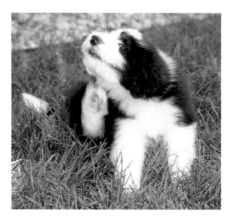

Flea infestation is the most common reason for dogs to scratch.

and between the toes. Pay especially careful attention to these areas. Ask your veterinarian about effective chemicals to eradicate ticks. Remember, all chemicals cannot be used on every species of animal.

Lice

The term *lice* is plural; one of the creatures is a *louse*. *Lousy* means infected with lice. *Pediculosis* is the term used for human infestation with lice.

Lice are among the few parasites that are extremely *host-specific*. Each species of louse lives only on its own species of host animal. Dog lice live only on canines; cattle lice live exclusively on bovines; bird lice live only on birds. Your cats will not get lice from your dogs. If your child gets human head lice, it was not from one of your pets; it was from a lousy little friend at school.

- Lice are easily spread when infested animals come into bodily contact with others of the same species. The common mode of transmission of dog lice is from the dam to her puppies. Cattle lice are spread from one member of a herd to the others. Human lice are spread among children by infected classmates sharing clothing, hats, or combs.

- Lice survive only a short time away from their hosts. They are seldom transmitted by contact with infested bedding unless an unaffected animal is introduced immediately after an affected one is removed. Horse lice can be spread to another horse by the immediate use of an infested saddle pad. If a louse accidentally gets on the wrong species of animal, it will not live long.

The eggs of all species of lice are called *nits.* These resemble tiny white seeds fastened to individual hairs of the host animal. Lice themselves are easy to kill, but it may take repeated treatment to remove the nits or kill new lice as the nits hatch. Your veterinarian will advise you as to which medications are appropriate for lice on each species of host.

Mites

Mite infestation of dogs is called *mange.* Canines can harbor several entirely different varieties of mange mites, only some of which are transmissible to cats and other animals. Mange mites are very small; some are microscopic, and some can be barely seen.

Demodectic mange in dogs is caused by the *Demodex canis* mite that lives in dogs' hair follicles.

Although the mites have been found on other animals (swine, humans) they are considered a parasite only of canines. This parasite is suspected when bald patches appear on the lips, head, and front paws of puppies. Victims of demodex mites itch and scratch very little. Demodectic mange is diagnosed only by a microscopic examination of a skin scraping. The long, thin, demodex mites are usually plentiful on each host, and easy to find.

- Small numbers of demodex mites are considered to be normal on canine skin. It is thought that a genetic or immunological disorder of some animals allows these mites to proliferate and cause clinical disease. Most cases occur in puppies from three to six months of age. However, even if you have a dog or puppy with demodectic mange, it will not spread the disease to any of your other animals, including cats and humans.

- Dogs with mild cases of demodectic mange often recover spontaneously. In the past, some severe cases of demodex were extremely difficult to treat, but modern drugs have changed this situation. Now most demodectic mange is controllable. Your veterinarian will prescribe topical or oral drugs if your dog is affected.

Sarcoptic mange is an entirely different disease from demodectic mange. The mite, *Sarcoptes canis,* is a round, eight-legged creature that lives within the superficial layers of dogs' skin. The most prominent sign of infestation with *Sarcoptes* is intense itching and resulting self-damage to the host. For this reason, all mites of the genus *Sarcoptes* are called "itch mites."

- Sarcoptes mites are host-specific, although they will live temporarily on species other than their primary host. Owners and family members whose dogs are infested with these mites often become affected with itchy red bumps that last for several days, even though the mites live on humans for only a few hours. The human disease, *scabies,* is caused by a different though related mite, *Sarcoptes scabei,* which will not live long on animals other than people.

- Sarcoptic mange is highly contagious among dogs. It is easily spread to other dogs by body contact. The mites cannot survive for more than 48 hours off the dog, so they are not spread by ordinary contact with blankets, collars, or other objects.

- Sarcoptic mange is diagnosed by microscopic examination of skin scrapings, but these mites may be relatively scarce on the host. When mites cannot be found in several scrapings, and when the host exhibits the severe itching typical of the disease, a presumptive diagnosis of sarcoptic mange is often made. If the diagnosis is correct, the administration of drugs lethal to sarcoptes mites causes the host's intense scratching to disappear very rapidly.

Ear mites are easily spread from dogs to cats, or from cats to dogs. As the name implies, this creature lives and reproduces in the ears of its victims, causing such intense scratching that the hosts develop open sores on the backs of their ears. The ears of affected animals contain an abundance of black wax; under a strong light sometimes the tiny mites can be seen moving in the wax even without a microscope.

Rabbit ear mites are a different species and do not thrive on dogs or cats, although they are extremely contagious to other rabbits. Rabbit ear mites are large enough to be seen with the naked eye.

Cats also can be affected with a different mite, *Notoedres cati,* which usually starts on the head and spreads to the entire body. These parasites are not contagious to dogs or humans, but may be spread to rabbits.

Sheep, cattle, and horses all are affected with species of itch mites.

Look for mites when your pup scratches at its ears.

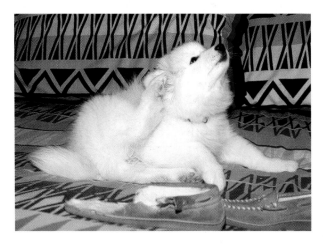

External Parasites Transmissible among Species

Parasite	Transmissible to:		
	Dogs	Cats	Others
Fleas	yes	yes	temporarily
Lice	no	no	no
Ticks	yes	yes	many
Demodex mites	yes (to nursing pups)	no	no
Sarcoptes Mites	yes	yes	temporarily
Otodectes Ear Mites	yes	yes	ferret, rabbit
Rabbit Ear Mites	no	no	no
Notoedres Cat Mites	no	yes	rabbit? fox?
Psoroptes Mites	no	no	hoofed animals
Ringworm M. canis	yes	yes	yes (humans)

Each of these mites has a favorite host, but each will live on other species temporarily.

Fortunately, modern drugs easily and quickly eliminate all Sarcoptes-type mites, including ear mites of dogs, cats, and rabbits. These drugs can be given orally, by injection, or applied to the skin. They also can be given to unaffected animals in the household to prevent them from contacting mites from affected pets. Your veterinarian will prescribe the correct medication and dose for each species.

Ringworm

Ringworm is a highly contagious skin disease of cats, dogs, and humans. It is caused by a fungus, one of many organisms related to yeasts and molds. The name "ring" worm comes from the typical circu-lar lesions that appear on the skin of the affected animal.

Microsporum canis is the fungus that causes almost every case of ringworm in dogs and cats, and some cases in horses and humans. In spite of the name canis, cats and kittens are the favorite hosts of this organism. Cats, especially adult cats, can be carriers of M. canis; they can spread the disease even though they may not have visible skin lesions.

• Ringworm in kittens first appears as scabby or crusty sores around the eyes, lips, and neck. If not treated, the sores may spread to the entire body. Cats and kittens with ringworm caused by M. canis generally do not itch or scratch.

• Your puppy, your kitten, and your child can all share this disease. Your child can get it from the kitten; the kitten can get it from an infected child. Older animals are more resistant to infection. Rarely do adult humans catch ringworm from kittens or children. Only occasionally do adult dogs become infected from either children or cats.

Be cautious when you obtain a new kitten. Take your new pet to your veterinarian before you allow it to have contact with your other animals or your children. Ask your veterinarian to examine the pet carefully with a Woods lamp, which may cause areas infected with *M. canis* to glow with a characteristic fluorescence. Ringworm infections in kittens are not always fluorescent. If your kitten has any visible sores, request a microscopic examination and a fungus culture of hairs plucked from the sore areas. It is not common to acquire a dog or puppy that is affected with ringworm. Be sure to ask your veterinarian to determine the cause of skin lesions on all new animals.

- Other species of fungus can cause ringworm in animals and humans. Horses can harbor *Trichophyton equinum,* which is spread by contaminated brushes and saddle pads. This infection is highly contagious among horses, very itchy, and can be spread to humans.
- Athlete's foot is a fungus infection that is contagious only to people. You can not get athlete's foot from a dog or cat.

Ringworm in dogs, cats, and humans can be treated with antifungal ointments, but is best treated with oral medication, often prescribed to be taken daily for several weeks. The medication penetrates the humans' or animals' skin and hair and kills the ringworm organisms.

Chapter Nineteen

Dogs' Manners toward Humans

Not everyone loves dogs. This comes as a surprise to the average owner, but many people have never owned dogs, fear dogs, or consider dogs to be "dirty animals." There is no legitimate excuse for a properly behaved human to be subjected to the unwanted attentions of another person's dog. Even though the dog may never, ever bite or scratch, it is the privilege of every person to decide if, when, and how he or she wants to relate to your dog.

The law is not on your side. A bite wound or a scratch is too often regarded as a life-threatening, lawsuit-causing event. Although a wound inflicted by a vaccinated, disease-free dog is unlikely to be more dangerous to a human than an identical injury inflicted in another way, the victim and the victim's family may think otherwise. You or your insurance carrier may end up paying the bill for medical or surgical treatment, even though the injury may need nothing more than a soap-and-water scrub.

In most localities, a dog that bites a human is subject to impoundment or quarantine even though it has been properly inoculated against rabies. In some instances, the offending dog is destroyed to satisfy the officials and the victim.

Teaching Dogs to Mind Their Manners

The Watchdog when Nobody Is Home

One of the strongest instinctive behaviors of the canine species is to protect its territory. Most adult dogs will react to the arrival of strange people by barking a warning. Barking at strangers is not bad manners; it is a dog's inherent right, even its duty, to bark at people who approach its property. Many dogs only bark; more aggressive ones will also snarl and threaten intruders.

Does a dog ever have the right to bite? This depends on the situation and your attitude about it. Under no ordinary circumstances should a dog

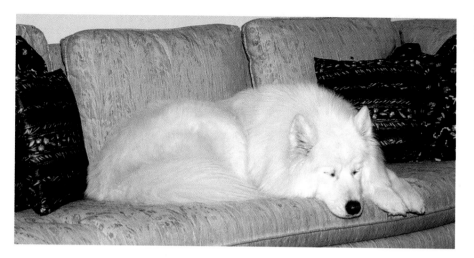

ever attack a human. No ordinary citizen should ever train a dog to attack; however, many people consider it the right of a dog to bite a stranger who enters its property without authorization or who threatens or commits physical harm to its owners.

In your absence, your watchdog should bark at all strangers. It should continue to bark until the intruders leave the premises. If your watchdog is outdoors, it must be confined behind a fence or otherwise restricted to your own property. Under no circumstances should your dog pursue an intruder who is no longer in your own yard. If it does, you could find yourself in big trouble with the law.

If you allow your dog to act aggressively when nobody is home, you must make provisions for those strangers who have a legitimate right to enter your property. Your watchdog must not be able to reach the mail carrier or the meter reader. If your dog prevents access to your mailbox or your meter, you will find yourself collecting your mail from the post office and paying higher estimated electric bills.

You may have a problem if your watchdog is kept indoors and is expected to challenge intruders in your absence. Many dogs will run from window to window, door to door, and damage woodwork and household furnishings as they jump and bark at strangers. If you confine your dog to one area inside your house, obviously it cannot guard the entire premises, even though an intruder may not realize this. Since most strangers limit their activity to ringing your doorbell, it is a good idea to train your dog to only challenge strangers at the doors. If you cannot prevent your dog from scratching the door in your absence, consider applying a piece of 1/8-inch tempered Masonite to the lower door panel. This material is very hard and resists damage from even the strongest nails. It might offend your decorator, but not as much as a destroyed door would.

The Watchdog when You Are at Home

Your watchdog has a different job to do when you are present. It should bark to inform you of the presence of strangers, but it should stop barking when you command, *"Quiet!"*

Some people want their dogs to remain at their sides when they answer the door; some people would rather their dogs lie down and stay nearby. If your dog is properly trained in simple obedience, you can make the choice in each instance. To keep the dog at your side, use the command *"Heel."* To have it lie down and stay in one place, command it *"Down"* before you go to the door. If your watchdog will not obey these commands reliably in every situation, it is not a real guard; your dog is merely following its instincts and not minding its manners.

Every trainer has discovered that there is nothing simple about "simple" obedience. The exercises may be simple, but the training is not. What can you do before your dog is obedient enough to obey *"Down"* and *"Heel"* when it becomes excited at the arrival of strangers? You will have no recourse but to lead the watchdog to an area in which you can confine it while you deal with the visitors. Of course, the dog probably will continue to bark while it is confined; you must tolerate this or you must teach it better manners.

To train your dog to *heel* or *down* in the presence of strangers, you will need an assistant (several different assistants would be better) who is not acquainted with the dog. Ask the assistant to ring the doorbell or walk onto your property while you enforce the commands *"Down"* or *"Heel."* It may take many training sessions to persuade your watchdog to obey you when its instinct tells it that it should guard your property.

If you have more than one dog, your problems will be magnified; each barking dog excites and reinforces the other. You must train each one individually before you can expect them to obey together. Start by training the most dominant of your dogs. Often the others will not display aggression if their leader does not.

Remember. Training never includes abuse. If you are harsh with your watchdog for doing what its instinct dictates, barking at strangers, you may unintentionally teach it not to bark at all. You could eliminate its function as a watchdog. Instead of punishment, inhibit its barking. Give your dog something else to do (*heel* or *down*) and make sure it obeys.

Good books on training will help. See Useful Addresses and Literature, page 134, for suggested titles.

The Friendly Dog

Most dogs will bark when anyone approaches their property, but most dogs are not aggressive once visitors have been admitted. These are excellent watchdogs for most people; they inform their owners that someone has arrived, but they never bite.

The best-mannered dogs bark briefly at the arrival of strangers, stop barking when told to, and remain at a respectful distance from visitors until encouraged to approach them. A well-mannered dog does not jump on visitors nor pester them for attention. Remember, some people do not like dogs, do not want to touch them, and consider any dog that jumps on them as attacking. "Oh, he won't bite," will not convince everyone.

Teach manners to your friendly dog exactly as you taught your watchdog. Set up several training sessions in which you admit people to your property while you control your dog's actions. Explain to your visitors that you are not ignoring them. You are teaching your dog to have good manners.

Dogs in Vehicles

Dogs should never be permitted to jump around in a moving vehicle, any more than a child should be allowed to climb out of its safety seat. If you are not sure of your dog's behavior, do not take it for a ride unless you have someone else to drive while you teach it car manners. Only after you are sure it will obey and stay down without correction should you allow it to go for a ride without another person driving.

It is not considered bad manners for a dog that is alone in a parked car to act protective of the vehicle. In today's society in which alarms and steering column locking devices are often used to discourage car theft, it makes sense to have a dog in the car to guard your property. If you choose to use your dog to guard your vehicle, use caution.

1. Never plan to leave your dog in the car for long periods of time or in unsuitable weather. The dog could suffer from heatstroke in the summer, chilling in the winter. If the dog is alone in the car for more than an hour or so, even the best trained ones may become bored and damage the upholstery.

2. Get a window barrier or open several windows just enough to admit air, but not enough to enable the dog to stick its nose out and bite someone. A surprising number of people will try to reach into a car to pet a dog. If they get a well-deserved bite, you may find yourself with a lawsuit.

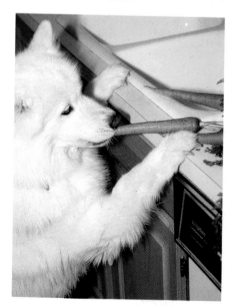

This Samoyed steals a carrot.

3. Even if you have a big, tough dog, *take the keys out of the ignition and lock your doors.* People have been known to "liberate" a dog left in a car, either as a prank, to steal the dog, or to steal the car. Thieves who see keys in the ignition can jerk a door open, wait until the dog jumps out, then drive away with the car. Once your watchdog leaves your vehicle, it will be confused by the strange environment and unlikely to bite.

4. Another reason for taking your car keys with you is that dogs may become excited when their owners return. Some dogs are excited when anyone approaches their car. If your dog jumps around and accidentally pushes down the door-locking buttons, you might find yourself locked out with the keys hanging in the ignition.

The Visiting Dog

Dogs are not welcome in everyone's home. Ask your host before you take your dog, even for a short visit. If you are not sure that it will be welcomed, leave your dog at home, get a friend to take care of it, or find a good boarding kennel.

Visiting dogs should never damage someone else's property. It is inexcusable to allow your dog to jump on furniture or lift its leg in your host's house. Unless your dog is exceptionally well trained, it is good manners to keep it on a leash or by your side for the duration of the visit. If you and your dog are staying overnight, consider taking an appropriate cage or crate in which to confine the dog when you are not attending to it. A dog in its own familiar crate will settle down in a strange place and allow everyone to get a night of rest.

Chapter Twenty

Humans' Manners toward Dogs and Their Owners

How would you like it if Granny countermanded your orders, allowed your children to stay up until midnight, play with the good silver, and eat only tacos and chocolate ice cream? What would you do if Grandpa permitted your children to grab sharp tools on his workbench and experiment on a table leg with his hacksaw? You would not like it at all. You have every right to object when relatives encourage your children to be rude, wild, and unmannerly. You have equal right to object when your relatives and friends encourage unacceptable behavior in your dog.

Dogs at Work

Seeing Eye dogs, guide dogs for the blind, assistance dogs, hunting dogs, herding dogs—all these have jobs to do. No matter how much they are admired, it is the epitome of bad manners to interfere in any way with a dog doing its job. It is not even appropriate to say, "Nice dog you've got there" to the working dog's handler; you can be sure the handler has heard the comment a thousand times. When you encounter a dog at work, stay out of its way. Step aside and allow the dog-and-handler team the right of way. It is extremely rude to shout instructions to the handler of a guide dog, even if you think the dog might need help. Of course, it is extremely bad manners to grab a sightless person by the arm at a crosswalk, an elevator, or anywhere else. If he or she needs your assistance, he or she will ask for it.

The Etiquette of Buying a Dog

It is the buyer's right and responsibility to discover everything pertinent about the animal under consideration. It is the seller's responsibility to disclose correct and truthful information. Neither party has the right to treat the other discourteously.

Classified Advertisements

Before you even unfold the newspaper, decide what you want to buy. Must your new dog be of a certain breed? Must it be purebred? Registered? Of championship stock? Of a certain age or sex? How about its health? Newspaper advertisements should contain enough information to enable buyers to tell if the dogs or puppies offered for sale fit their requirements, but too often advertisements are vague and incomplete. It is not bad manners to question the seller over the phone about anything the advertisement does not make clear. It is not bad manners to tell the seller that the dogs do not seem to be what you want. It is bad manners and a waste of everyone's time to go see a dog you have no intention of buying.

Papers. It is not bad manners to ascertain if the sellers of purebred dogs are in possession of the registration certificates and other essential documents. If the papers are "pending," it is not impolite to suggest that the seller contact you when he or she has them. Papers and certificates that are promised for later delivery often never arrive.

You should ask if the seller has veterinary certificates verifying that their dogs have been vaccinated or treated for worms. Sellers who give their own shots may or may not give the correct shots, give them properly, or use effective products. If you are not satisfied with an animal's medical treatment, consider that you will have additional veterinary expenses when you have the animal vaccinated again.

Price. Many classified advertisements do not state the price of the animals. It is acceptable to ask the seller how much the dogs cost. If you think it is too high, it is acceptable to politely state that the price is out of your range. It is not good manners to compare the cost to the price of others of the same breed, often offered in the same newspaper. If the dogs are priced much above the average, sellers are likely to justify their price by describing their animals' quality. They may state that they are champion-sired, show quality, have had extensive veterinary care, or have parents that excel in the obedience ring. It is up to the

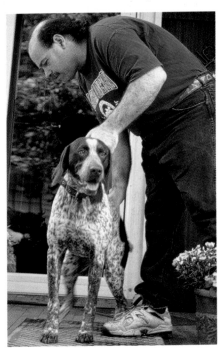

The owner must teach his dog how to behave.

Be a Real Dog Lover

Unfortunately, many people feel that they have to prove they are dog lovers by demonstrating excessive affection toward other people's dogs. Real dog lovers exercise good manners toward dogs that do not belong to them. Every dog lover should learn to be an RDL.

- RDLs leave other people's dogs alone. RDLs never coax someone else's dog to break position when its owner has told it to *down* or *stay*. RDLs never slap their thighs, snap their fingers, or whistle to reinforce an owner's command to *come*. RDLs never interfere with an owner's training by sound or gesture.

- RDLs do not encourage other people's dogs to jump on them or to jump on the couch to sit next to them. They do not grab or hug other people's dogs. They do not pet their host's dogs excessively nor do they talk baby talk to them.

- RDLs *never* object to owners' disciplining their own dogs. RDLs never say, "Oh, he's all right," when an owner tells a dog not to solicit petting from a visitor.

- RDLs never offer a bite of food to a dog without asking the owner first. RDLs never feed their host's dog at the table, even if the owners do. RDLs never give the neighbor's dog scraps when the neighbor is not looking.

- RDLs pet other people's dogs only when the owner has allowed the dog to approach in a mannerly fashion. RDLs give other people's dogs only a brief pat; RDLs certainly never initiate play action with other people's dogs.

- When RDLs see people with dogs on leashes, they might say, "Nice dog you've got there," but RDLs never pet or touch a stranger's dog without permission.

- RDLs never allow their own dogs to approach strange dogs on the street, just as they would never allow their children to approach strange dogs anywhere without the owner's permission.

- RDLs are respectful of other people's property. They do not allow their dogs to eliminate on their neighbors' lawns.

- RDLs certainly never tell dog owners how to train their own dogs.

buyer to evaluate the sellers' description. Remember, quality is a relative term. If you decide to pay for "quality," be sure you are receiving it.

If the seller refuses to disclose the price of a dog over the phone, you have the right to decline to consider the animal. Some sellers who will not tell you the price may think you will fall in love with their pups and be talked into paying more than you intended.

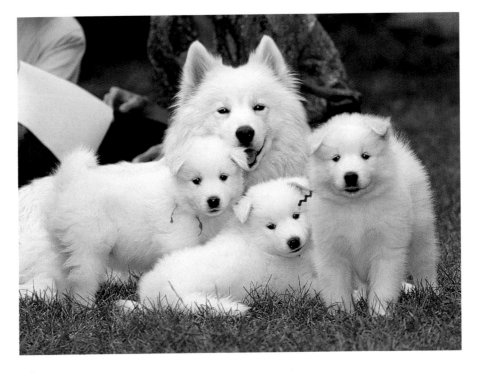

Samoyed mother and pups relax amid decision over new homes.

Inspecting a Dog or Puppy

You will probably go to a person's home or kennel to look at dogs offered for sale. Go alone or take one, at the most two, other people. Do not invade the seller's property with your entire family of children to play with the puppies. Remember, this is a business transaction, not a social occasion. If you must take children, let them stay in the car until you have determined if you want to buy the dog. Then, if the dog is over four or five months of age, it is polite to ask the seller if you may bring in a child or two to see how the dog acts toward children. If you are buying a younger puppy, you need not see if the pup likes children. Its behavior will be entirely determined by how you train it and how you train your children!

Health. It is not bad manners to insist that the seller of a dog or puppy guarantee its health. You do not need to take a seller's word that the puppy may be returned for a refund if found by a veterinarian not to be healthy. Get it in writing and agree to a reasonable length of time, such as ten days, for this agreement. If the dog is guaranteed against physical defects that may appear later in its life, this must also be in writing. If the dog is not as guaranteed, only you can decide if you are willing to accept a replacement dog instead of a refund.

Bargaining. If you decide that the asking price of a dog is too high, it is perfectly polite to tell the seller that you do not want to pay that much. It is not polite to try to bargain the price down, even though many sellers will invite you to make an offer. It is never good manners to criticize the seller's animals, nor to compare them unfavorably to others you have seen.

You may tell the seller that you have other dogs to see before you make a decision. It is terribly rude to ask a seller to hold a puppy for you and then cancel the purchase later. Other sales may be lost while you are making up your mind. You may ask a seller to hold a puppy only for a brief time, such as a day, if you really think you will buy it.

The Seller May Refuse a Sale

The purchase of living animals involves emotional factors not present in the sale of inanimate objects. Sellers have every right to refuse to sell a dog to persons that they feel will not provide a good home. The reasons for refusing a sale should be stated clearly and politely. There is no excuse for anger or shouting. All parties should part friends.

The Seller May Insist on Cash

If the buyer and the seller are strangers, it is not impolite for the seller to ask for cash or a certified check. It is certainly not impolite for the seller to ask to see some form of identification before accepting a check. A few breeders will sell puppies on time payments. It is not bad manners for the seller to get the terms in writing, signed by the buyer. If the seller agrees in writing to furnish the registration certificate only after the final payment is made, the certificate should be available for the buyer to inspect before the agreement is signed.

The Seller May Set the Terms of the Sale

Breeders of purebred dogs often sell puppies that do not meet their standards to become show dogs or working dogs. It is not incorrect for the purchasers of these dogs to be given the registration papers only after the dogs have been spayed or neutered. This agreement should be stated in writing. Other documents such as pedigrees and health papers should accompany every puppy at the time of sale.

Glossary

Please note that the following definitions set forth the meanings of these words as they are used specifically in this text. They are not intended to be full and complete definitions.

alter: to surgically remove the reproductive organs of either sex.

bacterial disease: a disease caused entirely by bacteria.

castrate: to surgically remove the testicles of a male animal.

choke chain: a dog collar made of a length of chain with a ring at each end. This collar is designed to tighten on the wearer's neck when the leash is pulled.

cutaneous larval migrans: a medical condition in which the larvae of roundworms migrate under the skin of a host.

dam: mother.

dominance aggression: the tendency of an animal to use force to establish itself as the leader of its social group.

external parasite: a parasite that lives on or within the skin of the host.

feces: stool or bowel movement. Also termed *fecal material*.

final host: the host in or upon which a parasite completes its life cycle.

food species: an animal upon which another species feeds.

free living: an animal that is not parasitic; the stage of life in which an animal is not parasitic.

headcollar: a device made of straps that fits onto the head of a dog. In both structure and function, a headcollar for a dog resembles the halter of a horse.

host: the animal upon which a parasite lives.

host specific: a parasite that can live on only one species of host.

ingest: to eat.

inherited: acquired through the genes from an animal's sire and/or its dam.

instinct: an inborn behavior or action.

intermediate host: the animal that harbors a parasite in a stage of the parasite's life cycle.

internal parasite: a parasite that lives within the body of its host.

life cycle: all of the stages of development of an animal.

microfilaria: the larval form of heartworm.

moult: to shed the skin or the outer covering of the body.

neurotropic: having an affinity for the nervous system.

neuter: to remove the reproductive organs; usually refers to the male sex organs.

ova: eggs.

parasite: an animal that must spend all or part of its life in or upon another animal.

parasitology: the study of parasites.

pesticide: a chemical that kills undesirable organisms.

prenatal: before birth.

prey aggression: the tendency for an animal to attack another animal that it considers to be a food species.

psittacine: birds of the parrot family.

puberty: sexual maturity; the age at which an animal is able to reproduce.

pupa: the resting or cocoon stage of certain insects.

sexual aggression: the tendency for animals to compete for mates.

signs: physical changes that indicate the presence of a disease in an animal.

sire: father.

social maturity: the age at which an animal is regarded as an adult by its peers.

social status: an animal's rank in its society.

spay: to remove the reproductive organs of a female animal.

submission: the tendency for one animal to yield to the dominance of another.

territorial aggression: the tendency of an animal to protect its home from invaders or those that it perceives to be invaders.

transplacental: across the placenta.

vaccination: a substance that creates an immunity to specific disease in a recipient animal.

vector: an animal that carries a disease or a parasite to other animals.

vermifuge: a drug administered to kill internal parasites.

virus disease: a disease caused entirely by viruses.

visceral larval migrans: the larvae of roundworms that migrate through the internal organs of another animal.

worm: a limbless invertebrate with a long, thin body. The term "worm" is often used to designate an internal parasite.

Useful Addresses and Literature

Books

Clark, Ross D., DVM and Joan R. Stainer. *Medical and Genetic Aspects of Purebred Dogs.* Edwardsville, Kansas: Veterinary Medical Publishing Company, 1983. Black-and-white and color photos, glossary, congenital defects. An excellent reference.

Coile, D. Caroline. *Show Me!* Hauppauge, New York: Barron's Educational Series, Inc., 1997. Answers many questions on the topic of dog shows, such as what physical qualities and training methods transform a dog into a prize winner.

Delta Society Working Group. *Learning in Dogs: The Principles of Canine Behavior and Learning, Implications for Training.* Renton, Washington: The Delta Society, 1995. An interesting reference with definitions of scientific terms involving learning and behavior.

Ellis, Vivian and Richard and Joy Claxton. *Make the Most of Carriage Driving.* London, England: J. A. Allen & Co. Ltd., 1995. Reference on training Dalmatians to accompany horse-drawn vehicles.

O'Farrell, Valerie, DVM. *Manual of Canine Behavior, Second Edition.* Ames, Iowa: Iowa State University Press, 1994. Intended for veterinarians, this text is very technical.

Overall, Karen, VMD. *Clinical Small Animal Behavior.* St. Louis, Missouri: Mosby Year Book, Inc., 1997. Another excellent, very technical text that includes the behavior of cats as well as of dogs. Stressed is behavior modification through the use of drugs.

Papurt, M.L., DVM. *Saved! A Guide to Success with Your Shelter Dog.* Hauppauge, New York: Barron's Educational Series, Inc., 1997. Includes one chapter on pet interaction.

Rice, Dan, DVM. *Dogs from A To Z: A Dictionary of Canine Terms.* Hauppauge, New York: Barron's Educational Series, Inc., 1996. More than 6,000 terms are defined, including everything from anatomy and medicine to showing and breeding.

Schlegl-Kofler, Katharina. *Educating Your Dog.* Hauppauge, New York: Barron's Educational Series, Inc., 1996. Emphasizes the importance of integrating affection and understanding into canine training methods. Nice full-color photos and how-to drawings.

Seigal, Mordecai, DVM and Faculty and Staff, School of Veterinary Medicine, Davis, California. *University of California Davis Book of Dogs: A Complete Medical Reference Guide for Dogs and Puppies.* New York: HarperCollins Publishers, Inc., 1995. A very complete work covering a broad field. Nice drawings, photographs, and charts.

Whitney, Leon F. *Dog Psychology: The Basis of Dog Training.* New York: Howell Book House, Inc., 1971. A good old classic.

Wrede, Barbara. *Before You Buy That Puppy.* Hauppauge, New York: Barron's Educational Series, Inc, 1994. Explores which dog best fits the lifestyle and personality of the prospective dog owner. Contains many color photos.

Organizations

American Humane Association
63 Inverness Drive East
Englewood, CO 80112
(303) 792-9900

American Kennel Club
5580 Centerview Drive, Suite 200
Raleigh, NC 27606-3390

American Society for the Prevention
of Cruelty to Animals
429 East 92nd Street
New York, NY 10128
(212) 876-7700

Delta Society
PO Box 1080
Renton, WA 98057
(425) 226-7357

Humane Society of the United States
2100 L Street, NW
Washington, DC 20037
(202) 452-1100

United Kennel Club, Inc.
100 East Kilgore Road
Kalamazoo, MI 49002-5584
(616) 343-9020

Some Sources of Dog Equipment

1. Call or visit your local pet store or pet supermarket. This is the fastest if not the least expensive way to find what you need.
2. If you cannot buy appropriate equipment locally, call for one or more pet-supply catalogs. Most of these companies advertise themselves as "wholesale dealers." They may impose a surcharge if your order is below a certain minimum amount. You may save money if you combine your order with the orders of dog-owning friends.

This list is by no means complete—many other catalogs in the United States offer similar material. If you request one catalog, you will probably find your name on the mailing list of several other companies.

Dr.'s Foster and Smith
2253 Air Park Road
PO Box 100
Rhinelander, WI 54501-0100
1-800-826-7206

Dunn's
1 Madison Avenue
Grand Junction, TN 38039-0449
1-800-223-8667
(Sells the leather prong collar)

J-B Wholesale Pet Supplies, Inc.
5 Raritan Road
Oakland, NJ 07436
1-800-526-0388

Jeffers Pet Catalog
PO Box 100
Dothan, AL 36320-0100
1-800-533-3377

**Max 200 Dog Obedience
   Equipment Co.**
114 Beach Street
Rockaway, NJ 07866
(Sells the "Flyball Competition
   Collar" with a built-in handle)

New England Serum Company
PO Box 128
Topsfield, MA 01983
1-800-637-3786

R. C. Steele
1989 Transit Way
Box 910
Brockport, NY 14420-0910
1-800-872-3773.

All these companies sell equipment such as the *Halti* headcollar made by Safari and the nylon fabric muzzle made by Top Paw. They also offer a huge assortment of collars, leashes, toys, and grooming supplies. If you can't find something you need, check the Internet under Dog Supplies.

Index

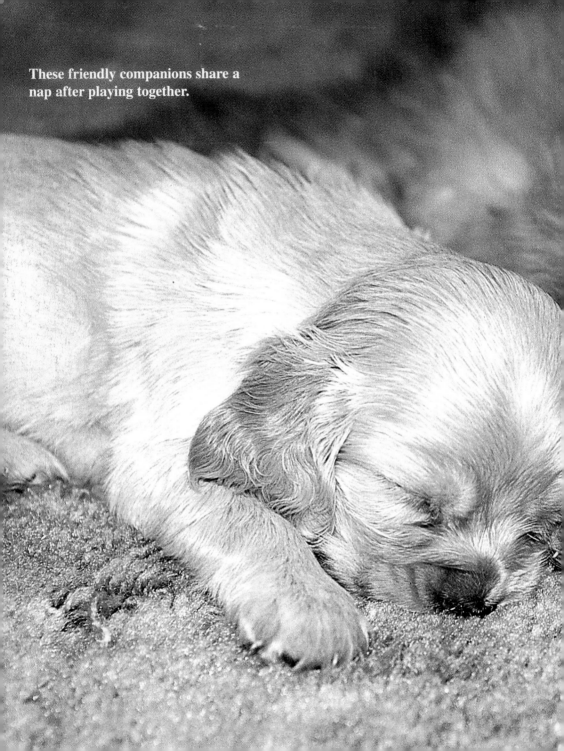

These friendly companions share a
nap after playing together.